KeeP
IT
MOVING

Motivation to Maintain an Active Lifestyle at Every Age

Raelyn Gregory RN

"Move It or Lose It..."

Table of Contents

Scientific and medical experts all agree that moving the body through physical activity is of   critical importance for maintaining optimal health and for .the prevention of many diseases. It is common knowledge that movement is good medicine. Exercise is crucial to supporting good health. Maintaining a physically active b ody has many benefits, including the ability to move about and participate in the activities you enjoy as well as the activities necessary required for daily living.

A physically, mentally, and spiritually well-balanced life is the best way to get the most out of life. Achieving this goal may easier said than done because there are so many other things involved. How you look, what you eat, where you work, where you live, what you do, and so on are all factors that contribute to your lifestyle. A certain amount of self-discipline and self-motivation are necessary to maintain a daily rhythm. As you choose ways in which to become more physically active, you will discover what works for you and what doesn't. We all have to accept that certain things are out of our control and there' no point in knocking ourselves out about them. Life patterns seem to go in cycles, so what works today, may not work tomorrow. We have to remain receptive and flexible to our changing physical abilities along our changing needs, and understand that leading an active life-style is a choice in an on-going process.

Because most body types are inherited and genes don't change, we were all born with a basic shape that stays genetically fixed. However, you can choose to be physically fit no matter what body you have received from genetics. Look around and you will notice that everyone comes in a wide variety of shapes and sizes. Eating healthy food , most of the time, and moving your body gives you the power to improve your body and become more fit, regardless of genetics.

It seems the whole world is obsessed with weight. Not a week goes by without another fad diet making the *New York Times Best seller List or appearing as the main feature on the nightly news. American currently spend over 40 billion dollars a year on quick weight-loss programs, diet aids, low calorie meals, spot reduction, and countless other so-called painless ways to lose weight. But there are two major problems with ongoing search to reduce. The first is that these programs are not intended for permanent weight loss, they are only designed to make the authors* rich by selling "quick-fix" fantasies. No one in their right mind would stay on a deprivation plan (diet) for longer than a few weeks. Although some weight is lost on these plans, it is almost all water weight and easily re-gained once the plan is ended. The second problem is that the information provided on diet and exercise is usually erroneous because it is outdated. New and exciting research is continuously being conducted in the areas of fat metabolism, nutrition, and physical activity. Thanks to the internet, the latest information on these topics is available to anyone with a computer, laptop, tablet, or iphone. But many American people still want to believe that rapid body changes can only occur through diet and deprivation. Unfortunately, there is no instant gratification; there is only mindful, consistent work towards the same goal.

Although more Americans are living much longer than their ancestors, most are not living more vigorously. In fact, many people live a large part of their lives merely surviving. The battle to get and stay fit can be won, one individual at a time. You can choose to regain a more youthful body and improve your zest for life. When you chose fitness you chose the ability to revolutionize your health, mental outlook, and general sense of well-being.

Our bodies are a unique and miraculous collection of cells, tissues, organs and systems comprising things like muscles, bones, blood, nerves, and fat. And of all those components, fat is the element that ends up causing us the most grief. Fat is responsible for a multitude of health problems from cancer and heart disease to low self-esteem and Type II diabetes.

Natural selection is a cold and harsh process that nature uses to cull out the weak and select the strongest of the species. This process goes on even in modern day humans. Today it will not be lions or wolves nipping at your heels trying to drag you under. The modern predators are obesity, heart disease, cancer, and other diseases of aging. Your best protection against disease is a physically and mentally active lifestyle.

In our forties and fifties our bodies switch to a 'default and decay' mode, and the free ride of youth is over. In the absence of signals to grow, your body and brain decay and you age. The keys to overriding the decay code exercise, mental stimulation, and reasonable nutrition. Life is either in the growth mode or the decay mode; there is no middle ground.

Everybody can improve their level of fitness, change their physique, and enhance their health in the process. One of the easiest ways to prevent muscle wasting due to inactivity is to give the body something to do. Research has conclusively demonstrated that exercisers of any age will increase strength, stamina and muscle mass. A federal government funded study on aging conducted by Tufts University demonstrated that the major symptoms of biological aging can be improved through increased activity. Strength, balance, endurance, and flexibility can be maintained or partially restored through exercise or through everyday physical activities that accomplish some of the same goals as exercise. What may seem like very small changes as a result of exercise and physical activity can have a big impact on your level of fitness.

However there is quite a bit of confusing information about what kinds of exercise is important as well as the best ways to do them.   The media is flooded with tons of exercise information; some of the information is accurate and some of it is complete nonsense. How do you know the difference? Read 'Keep It Moving' and you will be able to make the best exercise decision for you.

There are many types and ways to exercise. But the most important determining factor is finding the exercise you like and activity that you will consistently do. An exercise or workout program does not have to be formal or fancy.   Any physical activity that provides the body with enough movement to burn calories, increase circulation, and in turn helps you look and feel better is beneficial.

Aerobic exercise such as walking, biking, or running is the only kind of physical activity that directly burns body fat. For fat to be burned, oxygen has to be present, this occurs through aerobic exercise. At the start of exercise, your body uses carbohydrates for energy.

Are you feeling uncertain about your current level of health and fitness? Well, you don't have to wonder about these issues any longer. No matter how old you are or what shape you are currently in you can develop a more efficient, better functioning, fit body. You must believe some part of that state ment, or you would not be reading this book. The journey you are about to begin will empower you with the knowledge to feel great and look better.

Life is about being able to function independently, take care of ourselves, and to do the activities w e enjoy. Being physically fit helps you live your life to its fullest capacity at every stage of life. Functional fitness is most important as we age.

You can be fit at every age, but it does require effort and commitment on your part. As you now know from experience, fad diets, and short-term exercise plans do not work. Getting and staying fit requires a comprehensive lifestyle change and a willingness to focus on long-term goals.

There is no "secret" pill, "quick fix", diet, or potion that will give you the physique or the level of fitness you desire. If that were the case 45% of Americans would not be overweight or obese. Diet foods, fads, and fixes simply do not work.

Pinning your hopes to these "magic" solutions will not get you the fitness level that you desire. Thousands of companies have become rich and made billions of dollars on those who believe all they have to do is "swallow a pill" to get the body of their dreams. To be as physically fit as possible, takes a combination of eating well and some form of exercise. Having an active lifestyle does not have to be formal, grueling or boring.

Making positive, lasting changes in your body will take time, regardless of your age or level of fitness. Change is a gradual process, with no quick path to long-term results. Progress is built on a foundation of commitment and repetition of activities that bring desired results. There is a scientific term called "Expectation Theory".

In short this term tells us that the things we believe will happen usually do. If you expect to live a long, prosperous, happy life, you probably will. On the other hand, if you expect to have a decline in your vitality after fifty, you probably will.

There are a few basic things we must take into consideration before beginning any physical activity. First of all, you need to decide "where you are" and what your personal goal is for your individual fitness objective. For some the goal may be as simple as reclaiming the ability to climb a flight of stairs without pain or beginning training for your first 5K race.

As you begin this adventure, forget the whole concept of perfection. Perfection is an illusion, unattainable by all. It doesn't exist. As long as you are making an effort to improve your life, that is all that is important. Focus on progress, not perfection. The time and effort you put into yourself are an investment in your future. If we want permanent changes, we have to focus on the long term. With deeper understanding of what works for your benefit, you will increase your chance to succeed. Decide to stay active throughout your life. Commit to yourself. Give yourself time. Be consistent in your approach to reaching your goals. Get the support you need. Maintain your motivation. And above all else, don't give up. Believe in yourself and you will be able to "Keep It Moving" for life.

We will begin our physical activity quest by looking the health benefits of an active body and why it is important to build and maintain in Chapter 1. In Chapter 2, we will examine ways every movement we make throughout the day benefits us in some small way. In Chapter 3, we will look at "functional fitness", what it is and why it is important. Simple ways to find motivation to become and remain fit will be discussed in Chapter 4. Explanations of the importance of building and maintaining muscle mass will be discussed in Chapter 5.

In Chapter 6 we will look at how food choices affect your health and appearance. In Chapter 7 we will look at the value of vitamins in sustaining a fit body.

Chapter 8 examines ways rest restores energy and rejuvenates our bodies. Chapter 9 will look at ways to sustain and maintain our mental "fitness" and maintain our brains. And finally in Chapter 10, we will look at ways to optimize our outlook on life and satisfy our souls. We will examine the significance of loving your life as it is, discovering the beauty in it, and looking at small ways to make everyday a personal celebration. We will explore ways having an "attitude of gratitude" sends more abundance into our lives.

Life is a wonderful opportunity for continuing growth and development. Discovering unknown parts of ourselves is a lifelong process of unveiling strengths and talents we may never have been aware we possessed. As long as we are alive, we are in a constant state of learning. Whether conscious or unconscious, positive or negative, wanted or unwanted we are constantly supplied with information.

We have been given the blessing to choose the manner in which we want to live our life. We can dwell on the sad state of affairs and convince ourselves how it must be impossible to be fit and healthy, or we look at fit people and learn what makes them successful. Each one of us has the potential to reach beyond our current boundaries and achieve new goals.

The decision is, and has always been, yours. By setting realistic goals, creating a plan and sticking with it, you can achieve the fit, happy, prosperous life you envision for yourself. No matter whom you are or what you do, you have the power to choose.

This book is about your attitude. It is about your attitude about your life, your body, and who you are. It is a book about complete fitness: body and mind. You have to want to do the work that is required to get and stay fit.

Tough decisions will be required of you. Staying fit and moving throughout your life is a commitment you make to yourself. No one succeeds without giving up something.

We have all heard the expression, "move it or lose it". Nothing is closer to the truth when it comes to maintain muscle and our functional abilities. When you keep your body moving it functions like a well-oiled machine carrying you through your day to day life while you enjoy all the activities you love to do.

Remember when we were kids, we would run, jump, climb, and scramble around effortlessly? It made us happy to land a cartwheel, jump rope, or run a 50 yard dash until we fell into the grass gasping for air. As children, our bodies are primed for physical activity; every muscle, ligament and tendon is supple and receptive. As we age our desire to move diminishes but our body's ability doesn't have to. In reality, it is not our bodies that force us to slow down or stop enjoying the things we used to do. It is our conscious connection to our bodies that diminishes and makes us "feel old" when we really don't have to.

Chapter1.   Ignite Your Fire!!!

It is generally well understood that being physically active is complementary to a full, act life. As a nation, America has an overweight problem. Current estimates indicate over half of adults in the United States do not engage in any regular physical activity. As more and more children spend more time on computers, video games, and in front of televisions, more are likely to put on pounds. Our increasingly sedentary lifestyles are putting society at risk for serious health problems including obesity, Type II diabetes and coronary artery disease. An active lifestyle ignites our inner fire and sets off a chain of beneficial reactions.

An active lifestyle provides the body with a bounty of health benefits. In many ways physical activity can be thought of as the elixir of life since it has multiple benefits. Being physically active on a regular basis: 1. Promotes and maintains heart health, 2. Sharpens brain function, 3. Reduces stress, 4. Maintains or reduces weight, and 5. Protects against the development of Type II diabetes.

Regular physical activity strengthens the immune system which decreases the chances of diseases and illness. The advantages of an active lifestyle range from improved heart and lung function to better sleep. Using muscles helps build them which in turn, increases the metabolic rate.

Metabolism is the essence of what keeps you alive. Scientists define it as the chemical

processes inside living cells that are necessary for the maintenance of life. You are aware that you

have living cells in every part of your body; skin, bones, internal organs, and brain. Because all of these cells require energy to perform their specific functions, metabolism is ever-present throughout your body. Inside each cell are the powerhouses of metabolism called mitochondria. The mitochondria's job is to literally take the food we eat and burn it up to produce energy. When you're young, the mitochondria work efficiently, keeping you lean with minimal effort. Your body produces heat when you perform the simplest tasks, like walking the dog or sleeping peacefully.

But as we age, unstable molecules called free-radicals alter the function of the mitochondria causing our bodies to alter its "youthful response" to calorie intake. Put simply, metabolism slows with age and the same amount of food we ate a few years ago, is turned into energy less efficiently. So, even though you have been seemingly doing everything right, your metabolism still s-l-o-w-e-d down.

Research has demonstrated that as you get older, several occurrences ultimately lead to the insidious, middle-age weight gain. The

first contributing factor to the unwanted weight list is inactivity or decreased physical activity. As you

get older, you get busy, you fatigue more easily, and you don't make as much time for physical

activity. Even if you did manage to work-out for the same amount of time as when you were younger,

overall you're probably less active throughout the day.

Secondly, you eat fewer calories and eat at the wrong times. Although you might think

that eating less would help prevent weight gain, eating less actually slows your metabolism. When

you don't eat enough, the body goes into "starvation mode" to conserve the calories it has stored. Our

bodies are programmed with a very sensitive mechanism that will quickly turn down metabolism when

it senses fewer calories coming in. When you go too many hours without eating or drastically reduce

the amount of calories you take in, your brain tells your body to slow down which results in your body

burning less calories. Your body also starts to burn carbohydrates and muscle protein leaving behind

stored fat. Restricting calories also slows metabolism by reducing metabolic "flow". Simply put, the

metabolism does less work, which is an undesired consequence of extremely low calorie intake.

When you eat more and exercise, you increase the metabolic workload. Your metabolism has to

work harder to process the calories eaten which are needed to supply the body with the energy it

needs. So, consequently eating less and exercising less are two large factors in creating sluggish

metabolism and resultant weight gain.

Thirdly, with age, we lose lean body mass. With less activity, more stress, and fewer

calories, you slowly say good-bye to the firm body of youth. Even if you were never a muscle-bound

beach body, you were still programmed by nature to build and maintain muscle tissue. Muscle loss

doesn't just mean that there is no bulge when we flex our biceps. It also means that our metabolism works less because muscle uses energy in the form of calories and fat does not. Scientists have estimated that Resting Metabolic Rate (RMR), also known as Basal Metabolic Rate (BMR), accounts for 60 to 75 percent of the calories we burn and is highly dependent on muscle mass. In fact, 75 to 80 percent of your resting metabolic rate is determined by your amount of muscle mass. The more muscle you have, the higher your RMR. The less muscle you have, the slower the RMR. This fact is true for both, men and women.

The rate at which your body consumes and expends energy affects your weight and shape. Metabolism varies from person to person; you may have a faster metabolism than normal, or a slower one. Seventy percent of your metabolism is your *basal metabolic rate (BMR) and refers to performs it vital jobs, such as breathing, keeping your heart beating, and maintaining correct body temperature. How fast you use energy during digestion (dietary thermogenesis) and how quickly you burn calories during physical activity are the other two factors that determine your overall metabolic rate. I f you want speed up your metabolic rate, you need to change what you eat and the amount of energy you expend to experience a difference in how you look and feel.*

Every decade, your metabolic rate drops up to 5 percent", is according to Madelyn Fernstrom, PhD., director of the Weight Management Center at the University of Pittsburgh. Loss of fast-twitch muscle fibers, used in high-intensity, occurs notably in the aging process.
Even though we can't control our age or gender, we can manage the foods we eat and master our metabolisms.

As you age, if you don't take any steps, your metabolic rate takes a nose-dive every year past the age of 25. From the age of 25 to the age of 65, most people notice a slow, progressive loss of metabolic power that translates into added, unwanted pounds. Without taking some kind of action, by the time you reach age 65 you'll be burning 500 calories *less per day than you did when you were 25. Do the math; that's 3500 calories a week that are not being used or burned. 3500 calories equals 1 pound of fat. So you know what happens next, unfortunately we all do. That's right, according to this equation, if you let your metabolism slow to this level, you can expect to gain about 1 pound of fat per week while losing muscle mass at the same time. But wait, don't close the book yet, there is good news.*

Without regular exercise, muscle fibers shrink, or atrophy. According to researchers at the

American College of Sports medicine, unless we exercise regularly, we lose about 10 percent of our

muscle by age 50, and the rate of muscle loss only accelerates from there. Muscle as a percentage of

total body weight diminishes as we grow older, along with strength and stamina. Though some of

these changes are an integral part of the aging process, considerable enhancement in muscle tone

can be achieved with regular physical activity and proper caloric intake.

If you got up out of your seat and walked into the next room and back, a whole host of processes

would be activated throughout your body that would bring you countless health benefits. With just a

few steps you would start changes in your breathing, heart rate, and brain on top of changes and

benefits you would be getting by activating your musculoskeletal system. Even the smallest amount

of physical activity can lower your stress level and signal your body to release hormones that will streng

then your immune system and boost your overall health and sense of well-being.

It is worth looking at the physiological benefits of staying active that go beyond muscle strength and joint health. Let's look at the bounty of benefits derived from fitness. People who are physically active on a regular basis: promote heart health, sharpen and protect their brains, reduce stress, and protest th emselves against diabetes.

We will begin with the heart. The heart is a muscle and works better when it is made to work hard. Few people realize that lack of activity is one of the leading causes of coronary artery disease. Coronary artery disease is the name for heart related problems from angina to fatal myocardial infarctions (heart attacks).

Early in life the risk of a sedentary life style builds slowly. A recent report advises that children exercise regularly have a need at least 90 minutes of physical activity each day. People who exercise regularly have a lowered risk of developing heart disease.

Research studies reveal that a person who exercises has a 45 percent lower risk of developing heart disease than an inactive person. When we are exerting ourselves physically, we pump oxygen into our hearts, which expands the bloods vessels, allowing blood to flow more efficiently and freely through them.

Exercise also improves cholesterol and lipid levels, further protecting us from heart disease. Regular activity also stimulates the immune system to decrease harmful proteins that help cause plaque buildup in arteries.

The brain is another organ that benefits greatly from regular physical activity. At any stage of life, our brains continue to change and respond to new learning. Exercise assists in that process. In addition, exercise also helps prevent age-related decline.

Exercise maintains or increases muscle mass. Muscle is very active tissue which means it burns fuel even when you are sitting or sleeping. Your lean muscles are the "engine" of your body. The larger your muscle mass, the more calories you burn. If you lose muscle mass you will need fewer calories to keep the body running. Any type of muscle loss results in a reduction in your daily caloric needs. Because exercise can preserve and increase active muscle tissue, it has a direct impact on daily calorie needs. Having more muscle mass increases your caloric demands at work and at rest.

Keeping active and shaping up can make you feel like a new person. You'll feel less tense and better able to cope with daily stress. You will also improve the quality of your sleep at night and increase your energy level during the day. Being physically fit can help calm our nerves and allow for better quality sleep, and keep our brains sharp and ready for anything. There is no better stress buster

Being fitter means literally that It takes more stress, physical or emotional, to trigger the stress response. Exercise combats the damage caused by stress. When we exercise our bodies release soothing, hormones such as endorphins, into our bloodstream. These calming hormones are responsible for the wonderful feeling known as "the runner's high".

Engaging in any kind of physical activity will help you get fit and stay that way. Any cardiovascular exercise will burn calories, which will help with weight loss. It doesn't matter what type of exercise activity you choose, as long as you move to expend more energy than you take in, you will get leaner and fit. The key is to find some kind of movement you enjoy. Once you find what you really like to do for exercise, it's almost guaranteed you will do it regularly. Your metabolism will also be boosted in the process, encouraging your body to burn more calories faster.

At this point its really worth pointing out the biggest benefit of being fit is feeling better. Once you commit to regular fitness activity you will gain so many physical and emotional benefits, it will be hard to believe. Being fit can help you sleep better, help your clothes fit better, and increase your level of confidence.

Often the terms physical activity and exercise are used interchangeably, but they actually not synonyms. Instead physical activity encompasses all body movement, most notably the activities of daily living, which will be discussed in depth later in Chapter 3. Exercise, on the other hand, is defined as planned physical activity with the goal of increasing fitness. Any continuous activity is a form of exercise; although it is spontaneous, unstructured, informal it is still beneficial in maintaining a fit body.

Although modern medical advances and public health measures have allowed a longer life for many, not all are healthier lives. Unfortunately the conveniences of modern life have also created the huge problem of inactivity.

As a result this country is plagued with the detrimental effects of physical inactivity and the complication s of subsequent obesity. Cardiovascular exercise has been shown to increase serotonin levels in the brain. Exercise is a powerful, free tool to help you bring joy and a sense of well-being into your life.

And if those reasons aren't enough to convince you that exercise is good for you, here are 10 more benefits of exercise:

1. Exercise increases stamina and endurance for performing the activities of daily living

2. Exercise reduces stress by activating endorphins, creating a feeling of well-being

3. Exercise to reduce the risk of heart disease and stroke.

4. Exercise strengthens the immune system and thereby increases your resistance to illness.

5. Exercise strengthens joints and bones, decreasing the chance for osteoporosis

6. Exercise decreases your appetite by acting as a natural appetite suppressant.

7. Exercise increases the number of calories burned, and continues burning calories at rest

8. Exercise strengthens heart and lungs so they function more efficiently.

9. Exercise helps the brain function more efficiently, increasing mental acuity.

10. Exercise helps decrease blood pressure and cholesterol by altering LDL and HDL levels.

Exercise is a great mood regulator. We've all heard about the "runner's high, but a more accurate term for this phenomenon would be 'exercise euphoria'.

Exercise stimulates the production of endorphins which are neurotransmitters released by the pituitary gland. These chemicals induce a feeling of well-being and also alter nerve transmission in a way that lessens pain. Keeping active and staying physically fit can make you feel lke a new person. You will feel less tense and be better able to cope with daily life.

Chapter 2: Every Movement Counts

Physical Activity accounts for somewhere between 20 and 40 percent of calories burned daily. Th e amount of activity you do during the day varies and so do the amount of calories you burn on any given day. You don't have to be a runner or an athlete to gain the benefits of exercise. All you have to do is get yourself moving.

NEAT is an acronym for "non-exercise activity thermogenesis". It's basically all the physical movement of our lives that isn't planned exercise or sports. (Technically, it also isn't sleeping or eating.) It includes activities such as cooking, shopping, and even small movements such as fidgeting. It turns out that NEAT can have quite a substantial impact on our metabolic rates and calorie expenditures.

NEAT is thought to be one of the ways our bodies use to manage our weight. If we gain weight, NEAT tends to rise, whereas when we lose weight, NEAT often plummets, and people end up sitting more without moving as much.

As NEAT researcher James Levine puts it, "we may come to appreciate that spontaneous physical activity is not spontaneous at all but carefully programmed". Even standing as opposed to sitting can be beneficial, which has fueled the popularity of "standing desks".

You will learn that physical activity may be what helps keep you young. Day-to-day tasks such sweeping the floors, walking the dog, doing laundry, or yard work count as moderate physical activity. Any amount of physical activity is better than none at all. All activity counts. By adding just a little more activity to your day, you can improve your level of fitness in the long run.

A recent study from the *Journal of the American Medical Association showed that people that burned an extra 287 calories a day had a 32 percent lower risk of mortality as compared to those who were less active. Best of all, the authors concluded, "Simply expending energy through ANY activity may influence survival in older adults." We were born to move, and we die prematurely if we don't. What this study shows is that you don't have to be an athlete to get some movement into your life. You don't have to think of exercise in the traditional sense. All household chores count as exercise. Go for a walk. Mess around in the garden. If you talk on the phone, stand up and move around during the conversation. Any physical activity that burns calories is going to extend your life and improve the status of your health.*

You may actually be surprised by how many calories you burn through your usual daily activities An hour of housecleaning burns 200 to 300 calories, and an hour of vigorous yard work uses 300 to 400 calories. Even the smallest movements such as crossing and uncrossing your legs, standing up, stretching, walking across a room, and maintaining good posture all require energy. These small movements are known as non-exercise activity thermo genesis or NEAT. Whether you are walking around the mall, carrying groceries, or vacuuming the carpet, you are burning calories.

Look for ways to use your body more all day long. Any extra activity will help burn excess calories. To activate your daily routine try some of these extra "movements":

1. Use the stairs whenever possible.
2. Wash your car.
3. Take a short walk for your coffee break.
4. Walk around while your talk on the phone.
5. Park at the far end of the store parking lot, then walk to the door.
6. Dust and sweep around your front door.
7. Take up gardening (indoor or outdoor).
8. Take a short walk after dinner.
9. Clean out your bedroom closets.
10. Clean out your garage or storage area.

For many, the thought of exercise is a sensitive issue. Many people don't like to exercise, and believe me, I understand. The truth is that most of the time I enjoy exercising but sometimes, not as much. Through the years I have come to the realization that how I feel about exercise is less important than how it makes me feel. Because I maintain a consistent level of fitness, I usually enjoy the challenge of a good workout. Most days that I am off work, I workout first thing in the morning because it helps me feel good all day and I have accomplished my fitness goal for the day.

The word exercise comes partly from a Latin word that means to "maintain", "keep", and to "ward off". Exercise and physical activity really do "ward off" ill effects of inactivity. You realize that you should do some kind of exercise to improve your level of fitness, but the prospect of a formal exercise plan can be intimidating, especially if you are a non-exerciser.

But what most people don't factor in is that any form of movement is better than none. One of the most important reasons to do some form of exercise is so that we can stay functionally fit and able to perform our activities of daily living. Even though we burn calories sleeping and breathing, we have to expend more energy to achieve physical fitness. The calories you burn beyond what you need to live are completely within your control.

One of the easiest, cheapest, simplest forms of exercise is walking. Walking is something that everyone already knows how to do. Anybody can do it. As a matter of fact most of us engage in walking every day. You don't need special facilities or equipment. Even the busiest person can find time for a twenty minute walk. Walking is healthy, convenient, economical and probably the world's most underrated exercise. Walking also leads to cardiovascular fitness and lower blood pressure.

Walking inside or outside can prove to be very beneficial, when made part of a daily routine. Walking for exercise really works. Walking shapes you up. Walking strengthens and tones your entire body, including your feet. Walking burns calories. Walking burns fat. Walking uses a lot of oxygen and uses the large muscle groups which increase your body's fat-burning power. And if you pump your arms as you walk, you will burn even more calories.

If your goal is to lose weight by walking, its more important to walk longer than harder. Remember to walk at a brisk pace with minimal interruptions. The walk needs to be continuous for a designated amount of time. Since moderately brisk walking burns about a hundred calories per mile, if you walked an extra mile every day you would burn off the equivalent of ten pounds in a year. A recent study of out-of –shape middle-aged men and women showed that when they walked for forty minutes four times a week their pulse rate dropped an average of ten points and their VO2 Max (the maximum amount of oxygen the body uses during 1 minute of intense exercise. The higher the VO2 Max number, the greater the level of fitness.) increased 30% after 5 months. Safe and effective, walking programs have half the dropout rate of other exercise activities.

Walking is virtually injury free. Unlike running, jogging, or aerobics, which can produce an impact almost three to four times your body weight when each foot hits the ground, the impact of walking is only about 1 to 11/2 times your body weight.

Equipment needs are minimal. Make sure you have a good pair of running or walking shoes that are comfortable, light, and fit your feet well. Wear thick socks if your feet need extra cushion. The correct posture while walking will help you get the most benefit from your efforts. Stand tall, and don't bend over to look at your feet. Try to walk uphill and swing your arms naturally to increase the intensity of the walk.

Try to find other ways to "sneak" more walking into your day. Park your car a few blocks away from your destination. If you ride the bus, get off a few blocks early and walk the rest of the way.   Plan to Park your car far from the entrance of the mall, Movie Theater, or grocery store. Take the stairs whenever possible.

Aerobic exercise is any activity requiring oxygen that uses large muscle groups, is rhythmic in nature, and can be maintained over a period of time. When done consistently, aerobic activity trains the heart, lungs, and cardiovascular system to process and use oxygen more efficiently.

Therefore, an aerobically fit person can work longer and harder during a workout session than someone who is not. Whether your goal is weight loss or a higher level of fitness, the longer the time you exercise, the more calories you will burn. Check with your doctor before you start any serious workouts, especially if you have existing health problems, are obese, of advanced age, or have never exercised before.

Functional fitness is an emerging trend in fitness and health. Exercises are meant to mimic

activities of daily living to improve quality of life while also improving health. It focuses more on

improving balance, flexibility, stability, coordination, agility and endurance rather than strengthening

single muscles. Sure, a person may have bragging rights that they can bench press 400 pounds and

curl 100 pounds, but can they balance on one foot and lift something heavy off the top shelf in the

garage without losing balance? Can they sprint 50 yards after their dog that has broken off their

leash? Can they shovel snow off their driveway without throwing out their back or getting too winded

to continue?

Weight training is great for muscle tone, hypertrophy, and bone strength, but it is not the only

way to exercise. We live in a three-dimensional world, and traditional weight training is two-

dimensional; forward-backward and up-down. Weight machines make sure that your two dimensional

workout is completely stable; you are working on a fixed course. There is no wiggle room, even if your

range of motion differs from that of the idealized machine. At least with free weights you have to

stabilize the weights yourself. We still need to add that element of side-to-side, or rotation, to get a

complete workout.

There is more to exercise training than fitness, there is also function. Functional Fitness is broadly

defined as fitness to improve real-world physical performance also known as activities of daily living.

These activities of daily living (ADLs) are just that; they are the things that people do on a daily or

weekly basis. Some activities are home-based, like getting out of bed, bathing, gardening, walking up

and down stairs, cooking, lugging groceries, and housework. Some activities are work related, such

as computer use, truck driving, firefighting, nursing, and various other jobs. Other functional activities are related to hobbies, sports, and games.

People sometime have difficulty with normal life activity due to injury, overuse, or degeneration due to aging. Staying physically active helps us maintain the ability to remain independent in everyday life. Functional fitness is the physical capacity to meet real-life physical challenges. A person who has achieved functional fitness is capable of integrating different muscle groups and relying on endurance and full-body strength to perform natural, physical tasks. One who is functionally fit should not only be able to perform exercises, but should also be capable of real-life activities, such as carrying a heavy suitcase up a flight of stairs or engaging in physical combat. Functional fitness is used by the United States Marine Corps (USMC) to prepare Marines for combat. This type of fitness is achieved through functional exercise.

The concept of functional fitness differs from that of regular fitness because of its focus on integration, coordination, balance, and correct movement. With this type of fitness, the goal is for different muscle groups to work together in close coordination. Functional exercises are typically much more difficult than traditional fitness exercises, which often involve machines that don't require the performer to balance the body or coordinate movements.

Functional fitness and functional exercise are the latest gym buzzwords. They focus on building a body capable of doing real-life activities in real-life positions. Conventional fitness training isolates muscle groups, but it doesn't teach the muscle groups to work together. The key to functional exercise is integration. Muscles are trained to work together rather than isolating them to work independently. Functional fitness aims at improving general movement so that these movements become easier, freer, more adaptable, and more comfortable when done in real-life. The purpose of functional training is to help one perform activities of daily living with confidence and without discomfort during normal activities done at work, home, and play.

Bottom of Form

Please consider the following question: What good is having the biggest biceps in town if you can't climb the stairs in your home with ease, run for a bus without knee pain or lift a bag of groceries without hurting your back?

Functional fitness means that the goal physically active and staying working out is preparing your body so it can perform daily activities -- walking, bending, lifting, climbing stairs -- without pain, injury or discomfort.

"It's training for life, not events," said Jarrod Jordan, an advocate. At the Sports Center at Chelsea Piers in Manhattan, Mr. Jordan, 27, a fitness trainer, regularly puts clients through workouts that have them kneeling on wobbly, oversized rubber balls, racing up and down stairs and balancing precariously on multicolored yoga blocks -- all in pursuit of core strength, flexibility, coordination and balance.

This approach, which borrows liberally from disciplines as varied as yoga, Pilates, dance and physical therapy, is "very much the direction of the fitness industry," said Micheal A. Clark, a physical therapist and the chief executive of the National Academy of Sports Medicine in Calabasas, Calif., which trains fitness instructors.

"The average person today has goals other than, 'Can I tone up my abs or my butt,' " Mr. Clark said. "More people are coming in overweight, with injuries, knee pain, back pain. Even people who are gym-fit and lean have postural and muscle imbalances."

The whole-body regimen may be particularly well suited to women. According to Mr. Clark, "Ninety percent of women want to tone their buttocks, stomach and the back of their arms, but unless they straighten out the front of their hips, strengthen their abdomens and learn how to use the glute muscles they won't get the muscle tone they're after."

The remedy, functional fitness advocates say, is learning to use multiple muscle groups in an integrated way. This runs counter to the idea behind machine-based weight training, which was developed to allow bodybuilders to isolate single muscle groups.

"Your muscles may get stronger working on machines, but you're not creating synergy in the body," Mr. Jordan said. "With seated bench press curls, while you're working your arms, the rest of your body remains inactive."

By contrast, Mr. Jordan said, "functional fitness workouts challenge the body to work collectively as a whole, firing up the muscles in a sequential pattern."

In putting together each workout, trainers can choose from thousands of exercises, including more than 25 ways to perform a simple forward-facing lunge. The equipment includes physical-therapy staples like rubber fitness balls and yoga basics like foam blocks and balancing cushions. Mixing it up this way helps mitigate boredom and the exercise dropout factor that so often follows. "Yes it's more difficult," Mr. Clark said, "but it's also more fun."

Trish Talerico, 53, of Clark, N.J., a hospital administrator, began functional training at Chelsea Piers with the goal of strengthening her abdominal muscles for better back support. "You think it's going to be easy when you start but it's not; it's difficult," she said. "I can see each week that I've made progress. Things I couldn't balance on before, now I can. I think it's because I'm now using the correct muscles in the correct way.'

A perfect example of a functional type of exercise is the classic bent over row. As you do the exercise, you hold the weight with one hand with your arm hanging straight down, and then pull the weight up as your elbow points to the ceiling, finishing with your upper arm parallel to the ground. Because of the type of movement, this exercise that will build the muscles of the back, shoulders, the arms. Compare that motion to a nurse bending over a bed to transfer a patient or to an auto mechanic bending over to take a look at your engine. So anyone doing a bent-over row will find a carryover in things you do to function in daily life.

Functional fitness is achieved by practicing functional training. This is simply fitness that directly relates to whatever you do in everday life. Let's face it; many of our lives are causing havoc on our bodies. Being in seated positions all day, working on computers, driving in traffic, and the shoes we wear can have a dramatic impact on the function of our bodies. It is important to develop an exercise program which can work to offset some of these tendencies. An example would be to develop a gluteus and abdominal strengthening program if you are in a seated position for many hours per day.

Statistics tell us that 80% of the population deals with low back pain, and being seated for more than 4 hours per day increases your change of low back pain by up to 300%!! I believe it is important to note that many people do not encounter this pain while they are seated. It is when they are up, trying to perform a simple task which they have probably performed thousands of times (such taking out the trash) when their back suddenly "gives out".

This is where functional training comes in. In what is commonly known as "traditional training" an emphasis is placed on how much weight one can move while in a stable position and only moving in one plane of motion. How many times does taking out the trash only involve one plane of motion and how many times are you supported while you are lifting the trash out of the can? Probably never!

A functional training program is going to involve the appropriate flexibility exercises combined with cardiovascular training and resistance training. While performing the resistance portion, think of exercise which will mimic everyday activities. For example, lunges very closely relate to going up and down stairs; squatting is necessary for individuals to get up and down out of chairs; performing pressing and pulling motions with a cable machine or tubing will also require the trunk to coordinate movement between the upper body and stability of lower body which is essential in everyday activities. In addition to these activities, if your feeling nice and stable, try adding a twisting motion to introduce additional planes of motion or combine some exercise.

Many people are unfamiliar with the concept of remaining physically active to enhance everyday function. It is essential to our daily lives that we maintain functional fitness. But, you may ask, what exactly functional fitness is. Since there are many definitions of the term "functional fitness", let's look at several definitions.

- Functional fitness is based upon the person, the task, and goal. Once this has been established functional fitness must have elements of training that move the body in three-dimensions, utilize gravity to enhance moves, create dynamic body movements, moves should start in various positions of life (standing, one-leg, sitting, kneeling, supine, prone, side-lying...), and move in different angles & heights.

- Functional fitness can be described as the body's ability to manipulate movement needed to perform every-day tasks with the least amount of stress placed on the nervous, skeletal, and muscular systems. Your body will move and perform better when the skeletal system is properly aligned. This is commonly refered to as the Kinetic Chain. Poor posture can result in movement dysfunctions that may cause imbalances throughout the Kinetic Chain. This basically means that your body may start to move less efficiently and with greater stress placed on the joints and spine as well as the muscles moving with less coordination. Training programs that focus on improving poor postural patterns, core stability, balance, muscular strength, and cardio respiratory efficiency have proven beneficial in improving the efficiency of the Kinetic Chain. You can then start to train your body to improve in areas needed to perform and tolerate the forces needed to carry out daily activities with minimal stress

- Functional fitness is being in shape to successfully perform the movements you encounter during work, sport & life. I often contrast exercises that develop "function vs. fashion". Athletes & the elderly seem especially interested in developing functional fitness.

- Functional training is when your body has been conditioned to a point where you can handle your normal everyday physical activities with out causing harm to yourself. For example, if you are an at home Mom who really loves to clean and shop then you will need to do some functional exerc ises that will help keep your muscle moving not only strong but efficiently such as:
Squats- Cleaning the Bathroom
Lunges- Picking up the garbage or the kids socks
Shrugs - carrying the groceries from the store
Those are some Basic ideas on what functional training is and why it is important to train functionally during your workouts.

- Functional fitness can be looked at as practice for what our everyday lives ask of us. For instance, walking up and down stairs asks the body to be strong on the way up and very controlled and stable on the way down. Simple stepping exercises built into an exercise routine can help to get that much needed practice for when everyday life puts a staircase in front us

- Functional fitness is training multiple muscles, nerves and joints together to prepare your body for the specific activities and demands of everyday life. These activities include squatting, bending, twisting, walking, jumping, climbing etc. Our bodies need to work in a controlled and coordinated fashion to perform these movements effectively. Exercises such as squats, lunges, standing rows, and trunk rotations require different muscles groups have to work together rather than in isolation. Some of the important benefits of functional training include:

* helps correct poor movement and postural patterns

* improves flexibility

* helps prevent injury

* improves balance

* increases muscle and joint strength

- Functional fitness refers to performing exercises that closely mimic activities of everyday life. It is not often that we lie on our back and push a large amount of weight off the top

of us, therefore the bench press exercise would not be very
"functional." Some examples of functional exercise include:

o Standing cable press
o Standing cable row
o Squats
o Bench step ups
o Shoulder presses

- Functional fitness refers to how well you're able to do all the physical tasks you need to do each day. For example, if you're functionally fit, you can carry a bag of groceries without strain, bend down to pick up laundry from the floor without pulling a muscle, lift a child without injuring your back or even perform regular exercise. A large factor in functional fitness is flexibility - and staying active can help. Movement helps loosen up the body, keeping muscles limber.

Before beginning any fitness program, it's important that you get functionally fit first. This means that you should be in shape enough to safely and effectively perform everyday activities, like bending, lifting, twisting and walking. After all, if you can't reach into the back of a closet without pulling a muscle, how can you safely lift a dumbbell several times? But it's also important to stay functionally fit even after you've been active for a while to keep key muscles in ready-shape. These muscle groups include your abdomen, back and shoulders, and lower legs (quads, hamstrings, calves). Below are some exercises that can condition these muscles:

1. Stretches (hamstring, quads, upper calf, lower calf)
Stretching your lower leg muscles improves your flexibility as it helps your muscles and joints move through their normal range of motion. Increased flexibility can also reduce the risk for injury and prevent post-exercise soreness.

2. Abdominal crunches (basic, twisting trunk curl, upper abdomen)
Crunches help to develop a strong core, which stabilizes your body and protects your back, whether you bend over to pick up a piece of paper or a dumbbell.

3. Back and shoulder stretches and exercises (middle- and low-back stretch, arm and leg raise, shrug roll) A strong back and shoulders improve your posture and help you perform walking and running exercises safely and more efficiently.

4. Lower leg (heel raise)
It's important to strengthen your lower legs for activities like walking and climbing stairs because it reduces your incidence of shin splints, an inflammatory condition that can derail your workouts. Heel raises are ideal because they strengthen both your calves and shins.

You can do an entire series of these exercises in 10 minutes. You should perform them at least three times a week for at least one week before you embark on any aerobic or strength-training routine. Afterwards, weave functional fitness exercises into your regular workouts to keep these key muscles in shape.

This next sample series provides flexion, rotation and extension of the spine:

Still in the Sack

1. One Knee Hug (lying on back – hug one knee into chest – feel stretch in lower

back – other leg can be bent at knee or extended.) Breathe

Benefits of functional fitness include all the benefits of regular exercise, plus many additional advantages. One of the main goals – beyond preparing individuals for real-life physical demands – is to improve posture and correct improper body movement patterns. Functional exercises can break many of the body's bad habits and teach individuals to use all muscles in proportion, rather than relying consistently on certain muscles and not using others at all

This can result not only in greater strength, flexibility, and balance, but also in fewer injuries. Functional exercise tends to cause fewer injuries than other types because of its focus on correct movement. Becoming functionally fit can also relieve physical problems such as low energy, back pain headaches, and joint pain. Sometimes these problems can be completely eliminated. Some proponents of this type of fitness say it can also alleviate depression.

Functional fitness takes a holistic view of fitness. Fitness encompasses strength, speed, endurance and agility. It includes short, sharp efforts as well as lengthy ones. Most people have preferences towards certain activities or exercises - long distance running, weight training or sprinting, for example. Functional exercises cause an individual to work on their areas of strength as well as their areas of weakness, building overall strength and coordination. If performed correctly, functional training leads to better joint mobility and stability, as well as more efficient moment patterns. Improving these factors decreases the probability for injury. These exercises strengthen core muscles and stabilize joints - the key to a pain- and injury free body.

Chapter 4: Maintain Your Motivation

Many people think that trying to get fit starts in a gym. However, research suggests that the whole process starts in your head. To start thinking yourself in shape, stand back and look at where you are now and where you would like to get to. Don't worry about how many times you've tried in the past. There are many ways to move past the current perception of yourself and move to a place in your mind where you start to act and feel successful. Release your negative thoughts and focus on keeping your mind in a positive frame. Be clear about your goals and how you will stay motivated to achieve them.

The time you take to prepare yourself mentally can be invaluable. If you really want to become fit and continue to exercise regularly as a part of your lifestyle, you need to work from the inside out. Master the mind-body connection. Try to stay in the moment during your exercise time and when you are choosing what to eat. When you stay motivated and connected to your goals mentally, your body will soon follow. Having a fit body for life is your ultimate reward and it is within the realm of possibility at any age.

The conception of an event or an end point in your mind is the beginning of its existence. In other words, "What the mind believes, it can achieve". Without a clear goal of what we want to achieve, the manifestation of that goal is almost impossible.   If you don't know what you want and don't believe you can get it, you cant. On the other hand, when you have a clear picture of what you want to accomplish and a solid belief that you can make it happen, then your success is almost guaranteed as long as you make a plan for yourself and stay motivated to stick with it.

Trust me, if you use your mind and motivation to envision what you want to do, you will start making different and better choices to become what you see in your minds eye. Your mind is a very powerful force that can help you achieve your inner vision of your desired outer appearance. The body you see yourself achieving is ultimately the body you want and will have.

Focus on the new goal. Speak to yourself encouragingly. Tell yourself what you "can do" instead of what you "can't". Be careful of overstating any situation. Things are never really as bad as we sometime make them out to be. Every time you find yourself being negative, replace that thought with a positive thought about you. Learn to focus on the good and all that is good about you.

It is only by starting and maintaining your motivation to make some real changes in your life that you will achieve your fitness goals. The trick is to find ways to enjoy exercise and discover that eating h ealthy food does not have to be boring. I recommend that you stay focused on what you want to achieve each day. Mini-goals are a great way to stay motivated because you do a little at a time. Some small ways to maintain your motivation may include:
*Passing up the junk food aisle in the grocery store.
*Eating until you are satisfied, not stuffed.
*Moving a little more each day.
*Staying away from foods that tempt you to overeat.
*Finding positive magazines with articles and pictures that motivate you to continue.

Motivation may be your most vital lifestyle tool. By reading this far you have already starred to lead a more active life. Research has found that people who take steps toward any goal, are more likely to be successful because they thought about what they really wanted to achieve.

What do your thoughts have to do with leading an active lifestyle? Plenty. We talk to ourselves all the time, all day long. We can talk ourselves into or out of anything. We are constantly processing information from the time we wake up in the morning until we lay down to sleep at night. We give ourselves more feedback than anyone else possibly could. This silent conversation is called "self-talk".

Self-talk can be positive or negative and it can affect all areas of our lives, including health, finances, relationships, and our entire outlook on life. And most importantly, what we say to ourselves in fluences what we do.

Self talk is very powerful. It can make our outlook on life positive or negative. Self-talk sends the same chemical messages to your brain as experiences do. Your body believes your self-talk. Self-talk can support or motivation and life goals or it can lead us to self defeat. By repeating the same thoughts over, and over the mind actually comes to believe they are true. What you say to yourself is far more important than what is said to you. Negative self-talk is counter-productive and discouraging, while positive self-talk is encouraging and helps us reach our goals. When we engage in negative thinking we convince ourselves that the things we are thinking are in fact, true. Our bodies react to this negative input by increasing heart rate, shallow, rapid breathing, and stomach tightening. Negative self-talk creates stress in your mind and body.

We are our own worst critics. We have a tendency to be hyper-critical of our bodies and general appearance. Being negative about the image we see in the mirror will not change the facts. We only make ourselves feel worse which lessens the motivation to change the aspects of our bodies that we can change. We need to learn to replace every negative thought with a positive one. Changing this internal chatter is not easy but is worth the effort because the negative thoughts do not serve us well.

When we switch to positive self-talk, we convince ourselves that all things are possible. By focusing on positive thoughts we are able to believe in and see our dreams come to fruition. If you are truly motivated to turn a negative situation into a positive one, you will summon up the inner strength to accomplish the task. Through repeated, conscious effort positive self-talk will become the new inner dialogue. The benefits of , instead of saying positive self-talk are numerous and include; a heightened sense of well-being, less stress, reduced risk of coronary artery disease, and a longer, happier life.

The change starts with making yourself aware of your thoughts and the kinds of things you say to yourself. Then begin to make a conscious effort to change your self-talk from negative to positive. Choose the words you use carefully. Try to phrase things by referring to the present, not past or future. For example, instead of saying" I will never become more active than I am now", say to yoursel f, "I will be more active today". Talk to yourself about the way you want things to be now. Accept occasional setbacks as normal and understand that any kind of change takes at least 21 days of consistent practice to replace an old habit.

Motivation is a fundamental key to the success of achieving any goal. To truly get motivated about anything, you have to really want what you desire. Whether it's a new job, new car, or new lifestyle, your deepest desire has to motivate you to take action. Motivation is the inner power that pushes us into action. Motivation fuels desire and ambition. Finding and maintaining the motivation to pursue challenging goals requires an attitude adjustment. Attitude and motivation go hand in hand. A strong positive attitude drives motivation. Motivation is strongest when one has a clear vision of the desired goal and possesses the inner force to "make it happen". Motivation propels us toward taking the actions necessary to make the vision a reality.

We tend to act in ways consistent with our deepest beliefs. Self-deflating thoughts send messages to the brain. So, often our thoughts become self-fulfilling. Decide to conquer negative thoughts before they take root by changing them to positive. Simply put, you can talk yourself into doing something or talk yourself out of it. Be determined in thought.

Believe that you are the architect of your destiny. Create the life that you want and deserve. We are constantly growing and changing beings. Our attitudes and outlook on life needs adjustment with every change that comes into our lives. Be willing and open to seek and accept change. If you are determined to be more active, get strong, and stay happy, nothing can prevent you from attaining your goals.

Willpower is the one thing that most of us hold in our hands several times a day. It's the mindset that moves us towards or away from situations that are beneficial or detrimental to our lives. Willpower is more than good intention; it is accompanied by self-controlling action. Without willpower, there is nothing to harness your will and control your impulses. Using willpower to establish positive habits is a major key to adopting a more active lifestyle. It does carry power, but willing and doing must go together in order for any change to occur.

Willpower helps us change obstacles into opportunities for growth and development. That's where "If there's a will, there a way "comes from. If we decide to become more active we can let circumstances dictate our choices or we can press on regardless of what stands in our way. By preparing ourselves for the inevitable obstacles of life we can deal with stressors by looking at them as ways to strengthen our resolve and to keep moving forward.

In addition, the accumulation of small decisions carries us farther than any one decision ever will. Every day, every hour, every minute we are offered choices. Should I sleep in or get up and greet the day? Should I walk or drive? Should I take the elevator or walk the stairs? These seemingly inconsequential choices help make up who we are. When we realize the impact of every choice we make, we will value the small decisions as well as the large. As the famous Chinese philosopher Lao-tzu once said, " A journey of a thousand miles begins with a single step".

We all know that physical activity can be pure magic for the mind, body and soul. But how do you go from a sporadic, on again, off again exerciser to someone for whom being physically active is a lifelong habit, as natural and necessary as going to work and eating regular meals?

Here are 25 tips from someone who has been on both sides.

1. The first thing to do is to ask yourself: Why are you exercising? Are you trying to get in shape for an upcoming event? Do you want to lose weight, sleep better, increase your energy, gain strength, add muscle tone and flexibility, or just feel a heightened sense of well being? If the reason you are exercising has anything to do with someone else (for example, your boyfriend

says you need to lose weight or get in shape), you need a new reason (and, quite possibly, a new boyfriend).

2. Set goals. Set both a short term goal, to achieve in three to six weeks, and a long term goal, to achieve over the course of a year. Make sure your goals are achievable enough that they are not discouraging, but high enough that you have an incentive to tie your workout shoes each day. It is also important that your goals are specific and directly related to your specific motivation for exercising. For example, my main motivation for exercising is to consistently maintain my brighter mood and the calm, energized feeling that I get only from exercising, so my goal is to work out at least 5 days per week. My other motivation is to gain strength and cardiovascular endurance, so my other goals have to do with how long and how quickly I run.

3. Keep an exercise journal or log. Write down how your exercise is making you feel each day. How is your exercise benefiting your mood, energy levels, quality of sleep, weight, and so on? Do some exercises have more significant effects than others? Chart your progress in regard to your specific goals.

4. Take photos of yourself each month in your workout gear so you have a visual record of your results.

5. Make sure you are working out hard enough to release endorphins. Of course, you will want to talk to a doctor before starting any workout regimen, and you want to make sure that you are exercising at the optimum level for you, your body type, and your fitness level. I find that I am much more likely to continue with an exercise program if each workout releases those endorphins and immediately improve s they way I feel.

6. Advertisements for fitness products (especially athletic shoes) can be tremendously motivating. Purchase a fitness magazine and make an inspirational collage of images, advertisements and slogans that speak to you. Post your collage where you will see it each day.

7. Make sure you are using proper technique. You want to avoid injury, above all, so check with a doctor or trainer if you experience any pain, or if you are not sure whether you are doing a particular exercise correctly.

8. Join an online community, such as WeightWatchers.com or Ediets.com, which encourages you to log and track your exercise each day.

9. If you enjoy working out with someone, call a friend to help hold you accountable for those daily workouts.

10. Join a group that combines fitness goals with charity fundraising. The Leukemia & Lymphoma Society's Team In Training, for example, provides training to walk or run a whole or half marathon, or to participate in a triathlon or 100 mile bike ride, all while raising money for a good cause.

11. If you prefer to work out alone, give yourself something fun to do while you exercise. Find some good heart pumping music or listen to books on tape. A suspenseful audiobook may be all you need to get on those running shoes each day.

12. Identify the excuses you like to use and have a ready made response. If time is an issue, make sure your workout clothes are ready to go. If you have young children, get a good jogging stroller or set up a babysitting swap with another mom in your neighborhood: you can watch her children while she works out and vice versa.

13. Make sure you have the right gear, which can make all the difference in the comfort level of your workout. A good pair of shoes is essential. And weather resistant clothing or a membership to an indoor gym can help you fight off your own excuses when weather conditions are less than ideal.

14. Once you find an exercise that you particularly enjoy, do a Google search to find out more about any coaches or specialists that may be able to provide inspiration or special training, either through tapes, books, or online resources. If you are a runner, for example, check out JohnBingham.com.

15. Recognize that your will to exercise is going to fluctuate, and exercise anyway. Sometimes it helps if I promise myself that I can stop my workout after 10 minutes if I still want to. At that point, I'm usually feeling so much better that I finish the workout.

16. Place a giant star on your calendar each day to indicate that you completed your workout. These visual rewards can be so motivating.

17. Change your routine as you reach new goals. Add zest to your workout and avoid the exercise plateau by increasing the intensity or the duration of your workout, or by trying a new workout or sport.

18. Hire a trainer. If you are in an exercise rut, consider consulting with a personal trainer for a session or two. You will learn new techniques and find fresh motivation, as well.

19. Try not to take more than one day off at a time. I have found this really important to avoid losing valuable momentum. If I take two days off, it becomes very easy to take another day, and then another day. That means that if your workout is only part of your weekday routine, weave it into your weekend routine, too.

20. Be gentle with yourself. If you miss a workout or two or three, get right back to your regular schedule. You will feel better instantly.

21. Choose an exercise that you are likely to do each day. Some experts say that walking is the best exercise simply because it is something that is easy to do on a continual basis. There is no need for special equipment, and you can do it absolutely anywhere.

22. If you are walking or running, get a good pedometer to help you track your progress.

23. Schedule your daily exercise on your to do list and in your planner. Think of it as simply something you need to do before your head hits the pillow.
24. Give yourself simple rewards. It is generally best if these rewards are not edible, since a food reward can be a tad demoralizing after you have just worked to burn so many calories in a workout. For long term goals, treat yourself to a new pair of athletic shoes or other fitness equipment. For short term goals, consider a new fitness magazine, workout video, or simply fresh flowers for the dining room table.
25. Try to think of physical activity and /or exercise as something you do for yourself: a gift you give yourself, a way to stay balanced and focused, and time when you can be alone with your thoughts.

Chapter 5: Make Some Muscle

Muscle tissue is worth its weight in gold. Our muscles, when they are strong, well nourished, and used regularly, are what power us through life. They lift us up and propel us forward. Muscles need to be used and to be used on a regular basis. That is why movement and muscle go hand in hand. If we don't use our muscles, they atrophy which means they shrink in size and function.

Muscle moves 206 bones in your body and gives your physique a firm, desireable appearance. Firm muscles are attractive and help to lift other tissue that might otherwise sag. Unfortunately, as muscles age, they lose cells. Along with muscle cell loss comes a corresponding loss in firmness and body shape. Existing muscle cells shrink and become less contractile and less flexible, making them more susceptible to strains and pulls. The good news is that muscle can be build or maintained with very minimal effort. . Start an exercise program designed to build and maintain adequate muscle tissue to fuel your body's around-the-clock fat burning mechanism, also known as your metabolism.   It really is possible to add muscle while you lose fat.   One of the main objectives of any over-50 fitness program is to actually *gain some muscle tissue. With each decade of life after young adulthood, the average American loses 6.6 pounds of lean-body mass. Many people who become increasingly overweight after middle age assume that their problem is too much fat. But research has demonstrated that the actual problem is a combination of too much fat and too little lean-body mass, particularly muscles. Fa t and muscle do not share the same metabolism; comparatively, fat is much more inactive. It serves as an energy-storage tissue, while muscle is an energy-spending tissue. Lean muscle tissue is extremely metabolically active, and additional muscle will ultimately increase around-the-clock fat burning.*

In a nutshell, strength training works because making muscles fires up your metabolism and keeps your body running at its fat-burning best. For every pound of muscle you have on your body, you burn between 30 and 50 calories a day, even when you are sleeping. Over time, muscle-metabolism gains can add up to fat loss. Be aware that lean tissue is so much denser than fatty tissue; overall weight loss is an inaccurate gauge of real progress. Consider this: If you gained 3 pounds of muscle and burn 40 additional calories per pound, you could burn an additional 120 calories per day, or 3600 calories per month. At that rate, those 3 pounds of muscle would burn off 12 pounds over the course of a year. Adding muscle tissue will make you stronger and give you a leaner appearance although you may, in fact, actually weigh more. If you are really weight conscious that means you will have to readjust your ideas about "weight" and judge your progress by how you look and feel. So, don't become a slave to your bathroom scale, it won't accurately reflect changes in body composition.

Muscle is valuable for many reasons besides making the body look lean and toned. Muscle is very active tissue; that means it burns fuel even when you are sitting or sleeping. Think of your lean muscle tissue as your body's engine. The larger the engine, the more gas it burns. The larger your muscle mass, the more calories you burn. When you lose muscle tissue, you need fewer calories to keep the body moving which reduces your daily caloric needs.

In terms of metabolic activity, pound for pound, muscle is the hardest working tissue in bodies. In fact, 1 pound of muscle burns about 35 calories a day, whereas a pound of fat burns only 2 cal It takes more calories to build, maintain, and repair muscle tissue than the same amount of every other tissue in the body. And because we possess many more pounds of muscle than any other tissue type, the vast majority of our calorie expenditure goes to sustaining our muscles. This fact is true even if you are mostly sedentary. In fact, if you are mostly sedentary, any slight increase in muscle activity can greatly increase calorie use and fat-burning.

If you are active, very modest increases in muscle mass will accomplish the same goal. Basically, the more muscle you have the more calories you burn. The more muscle you have the higher your resting metabolic rate and the more calories you will burn over time, even at rest. You don't have to spend hours in the gym lifting heavy weights to reap the benefits of a revved up metabolism, a little extr a muscle goes along way.

The old adage "use it or lose it" is especially true when it comes to maintaining a fit body. Adults who don't exercise regularly will typically lose between five to seven pounds of muscle every decade. To put this fact into perspective, a five pound muscle loss translates to about 250 fewer calories burned each day which can add up to over 25 pounds gained in one year.

Studies reveal that between the ages of 20 and 30, without weight bearing exercise, we begin to lose muscle. As we age, the rate at which we lose muscle seems to decrease slightly. As we lose muscle, our metabolic rate slows down, which means we burn are burning fewer calories. This change in metabolism generally leads to a gain in fat. Muscle is denser and takes up less space than fat. Gerontologists have found that muscle is much more responsible for the body's overall vitality than most people, including most doctors ever, ever supposed. Based on their research, the Tufts investigators found that muscle mass, along with strength, is critical and that by building muscles late in life, old people can significantly rejuvenate their whole physiology. Since the rate at which you lose lean-body mass accelerates after age 45, the researchers concentrated on full-scale exercise programs for the 45+ age groups, reversing the social programming that says vigorous physical activity belongs to the young. Previously, a decline in muscle strength was considered unavoidable, and expected with increasing age. The Tufts group conclusively proved that a decline in muscle strength was not only *not inevitable, but also reversible.* *Twelve men between the ages of 60 and 72 were put on a regular supervised weight training program three times a week for three months. They were asked to train at 80 percent of their "repetition maximum", the heaviest weight they could lift at one try. At the end of the* experiment, the men's strength had increased dramatically, the size

of their quadriceps had doubled, and their hamstrings had nearly tripled in size. Milder weight training

programs for **people over 95 proved equally successful. My point is, the idea of "taking it**

easy" as we get older needs to be reexamined. Clearly, that idea is really not the best for your

body or your brain.   My suggestion to you and plan for myself, is to remain at the most

youthful level of functioning possible.

Physical fitness is very closely linked to one's general sense of well-being; most people who work

out regularly report feeling younger and better about themselves overall.   The main objective of

many fitness programs is to gain muscle tissue. When you start an exercise program that includes

activities designed to build and maintain muscle tissue, you are also helping your body boost

metabolism and calorie-burning. Fat and muscle do not share the same metabolism. Fat is inactive

and serves as energy-storing tissue. On the other hand, muscle is an energy spending tissue.

When you build and develop muscles, they burn more calories. Lean muscle tissue is extremely

metabolically active so having muscle will more ultimately increase around the clock fat burning.

With each decade of life after young adulthood, the average adult loses 6.6 pounds of lean body

mass. Many people who become increasingly overweight after middle age assume the problem with

their bodies is too much fat. But research has demonstrated that the actual problem is a combination

of too much fat and too little lean body mass, particularly muscle tissue.

Making muscles fires up your metabolism and keeps your body functioning more efficiently at fat
burning. To maintain every pound of muscle you have, you burn between 30 and 50 calories a day,
even while sleeping. Be aware that lean muscle tissue is much more dense than fat, so it weighs
more. Therefore the number reflected on a scale is not necessarily an accurate measurement of real
progress. If you gained 3 pounds of muscle and burn an additional 40 calories

Weight is not the only gauge of health and fitness. Most personal trainers will tell you not to

worry about the scale anyway, but to focus on the way your clothes fit. Instead of fixating on pounds, getting fit should be the goal. You can be in excellent cardiovascular condition and still have a thick

waist and wide hips. Maybe your natural metabolic program tells your body to store extra fat and you c

an't lose it no matter how hard you try. Realize that genetically your body is predisposed to certain

characteristics. You can capitalize on your attributes and become fit. People of any age who are

physically fit naturally feel and look better. Accentuate the best of your inherited traits by adding exercise and healthful eating. The remainder of this chapter will be dedicated to exercises involving the three areas people surveyed named as the most troublesome parts of their physiques as they age; the abdomen, thighs and buttocks (also known as potbelly, thunder thighs, and flabby butt). In order to keep from overwhelming you as you start your new exercise program, I am going to limit each area to five exercises. You can always add more to your personal program as you get more into the habit of exercising, but for now I don't want to discourage you, or scare you off before you even begin so we will start with just five.

Your abdominal muscles confine your internal organs like a snug girdle. But aging, lack of exercise, and a poor diet can quickly transform the abdominal area into a spreading, overgrown pouch. Also known as the "middle-age spread", this was the number one area of concern listed by both genders after age 50. The trouble is we don't routinely tax our abs very much during the course of a day. If we worked them harder, or more often, or both, they would tighten up, get stronger, and our abdominal area wouldn't protrude. Anything that you can do to tighten your abdominal muscles will help hold in your stomach. Your abs consists of four muscles, all of which shape your midsection:

- The rectus abdominus (upper and lower), a vertical muscle that run from your rib cage to your pubic bone:
- The transverse abdominus, the deepest ab, which runs horizontally from your ribs to your hips:
- The external oblique, a broad, thin muscle that runs diagonally from your ribs to your hip:
- The internal oblique muscle, which runs along the front and sides of your torso.

To slim the abdominal area, you need a program of exercises that deliberately works the abs, especially the upper, lower, and the obliques. The abdominal muscles are an excellent group to start with because they respond very quickly to exercise. Compared to the buttocks, thighs, or other muscle groups, the abs get stronger pretty quickly. Now bear in mind, that strong doesn't automatically mean flat. In order to get the entire benefit of ab work, you will have to limit the amount of fat that you consume in your diet. Sorry, but that's the deal. You can expect to have less fat around your abdomen unless you pay attention to what you eat and put less fat into your mouth.

The workouts that follow produce results because they use the principle of *overload*. *Overloading any muscle occurs either by increasing the number of repetitions of an exercise or by incre asing intensity which means doing the same number of repetitions but adding weights to make the exercise harder. If you are new to exercise, start slow and build reps and intensity as you become stronger. Trying to do too much in the beginning will result in injuries and set-backs. Form is much more important than the number of repetitions or the amount of weight that you use. Proper form will get you the results that you want and prevent you from getting hurt. If you are consistent and stick to the minimum 3-day a week exercise plan, you should start to feel a difference in your midsection after about two weeks. By four weeks, you should see some tightening or slight changes in contour. And by six weeks you should look and feel toned. I will provide you with a "workout" version and an "everyday" version of all the exercises that I recommend so that you can wok the same muscles in your daily life. Here are some more tips to help you succeed and get the results that you are looking for:*

1. **Work your entire body. Despite what you've heard, aerobic exercise can tone your muscles to some degree depending on the type and duration of the exercise. Most people do aerobic exercise for the cardiovascular effects, but research has shown that 20-30 percent of the effort carries over to strengthen and tone muscles.**

2. **Start Easy. Five to 10 repetitions should be the maximum for the first 2-4 weeks. Listen to your body and you will know when it is time to advance.**

3. **Be Consistent, Be Realistic, and Be Patient.** Next to performing the exercises correctly, exercising regularly is key. Don't expect results overnight. As mentioned earlier, you need to do the exercises at least 3 to 4 times a week for least 6 weeks to notice in real difference in your body. wasn't built in a day, your body didn't get this way in a day, and it's going to take more than a day to fix it. You get the point. No miracle fixes here, that's a promise I made from the start. You have to put in the work to get the reward.

4. **Be Mindful of What you are Eating.** I'm not going to harp on this subject, but I want to make sure that you understand the exercise/food connection. No matter how many

crunches you do, if you are eating a high fat diet, your abdomen and your whole body will tell the story.

5. Keep It Moving. No toning exercises alone are going to sculpt your entire body, they will help but no one way will do the entire job. Combining aerobic type exercise (like walking) with any other type of workout will help your body by burning calories which helps get rid of excess weight all over.

6. Do the exercises correctly to avoid injury. This is especially important if you are new to working out or haven't worked out for a long time. Don't rush through the exercises. Feel the muscles that are being worked.

7. Keep your movements tight and controlled. Don't swing your way through or let momentum do the work. Use the muscle group that you are working. Visualize that muscle in your mind.

8. Make yourself Comfortable. Wear comfortable clothes and shoes. Train yourself to look forward to your work-out session as a kind of personal escape where you do something good for you.

Here are the top 5 abdominal exercises I recommend for beginning abdominal training to achieve the best results in a shorter period of time. Some are compound exercises which work two or more body part at once which also increases calorie burn. I will describe how to do each exercise, give tips on performing each, describe the "everyday" version of the exercise, describe the muscle group worked, and prescribe the intensity at which the exercise should be done. Hopefully you will find this format easy to follow and user-friendly. I incorporate this group of exercises into my work-out routine, no matter which routine I happen to be doing at the time. I know they work.

The 'KEEP IT MOVING' Abdominal Series:

Exercise 1: Knee-Up Crunches: Lie on your back with knees parallel to the floor. Fold your arms across your chest. Using the muscles of your upper abs, lift your shoulders and upper back off the floor. Hold for 2 seconds then slowly lower yourself to starting position. Do three sets of 5-10 repetitions.

Muscles Worked: Upper Abs.

TIPS: Make sure that your shoulders lift off the floor. Don't use momentum to do the move. Keep the small of your back flat against the floor. Raise your shoulders during the exhale and keep your abdomen flat.

Everyday Version: You can simulate this exercise while lying on the floor with your legs up on a chair, or sofa.

Exercise 2: Side Bends: Stand with your knees slightly bent, feet shoulder-width apart, hands behind your head with elbow extended out to the sides. Bend to your right side in a slow controlled movement, bringing your right elbow toward your right knee. Return to standing position and repeat the bend to the left side. One bend to each side is counted as one rep. Repeat the exercise until you have finished your repetitions. Do three sets of 5-10 repetitions.

Muscles Worked: Obliques

TIPS: Do the exercise in a slow controlled movement throughout the full range of motion. Use your oblique muscles, not momentum, to perform the repetitions. Don't lean forward as you do the move, try to keep your body centered.

Everyday Version: Stand with your feet comfortably apart in a semi-squat position with your hands behind your head and your elbows extended out. Bend to one side about 20 to 30

degrees and hold for 5 seconds, and then relax. Repeat on opposite side. Alternate sides until

reps completed.

Exercise 3: The Bicycle: Lie on your back with your feet flat on the floor with your knees bent.

Clasp your hand behind your head with elbows out to the sides. Simultaneously lift your

head and shoulders off the floor as you extend the left leg and rotate your right elbow to your

left knee, then repeat the exercise in the opposite direction. Try to keep your abdomen flat

and exhale as you twist. These exercises are really hard but they get quick results, so try to do

3-7 reps until you become stronger.

Muscles Worked: Upper, obliques, and lower abs

TIPS: Do not pull on your head and neck with your arms while lifting and rotating. Do not twist

too far. Don't use momentum when alternating sides. As you turn your torso, keep your abs

contracted throughout the movement.

Everyday Version: While standing at your kitchen sink or waiting in line, fold your arms,

contract your abs, and rotate your body slowly to one side in a slow controlled motion. Hold

for 5 seconds, and then repeat to the opposite side.

Exercise 4: Reverse Curls: Lie flat on your back with your hands behind your head and

elbows out. Raise your legs with knees bent to a 90 degree angle. Using your lower abs, raise

your hips toward your ribs and hold for a count of 2. Then lower your hips, keeping your abs

contracted until your hips touch the floor. Do three sets of 5-10 reps.

Muscles Worked: Lower abs

TIPS: Don't rock or use momentum to perform the curl. Keep constant tension on your abs during the exercise. Don't raise your head and neck off the floor.

Everyday Version: While sitting, you can do pelvic tilts that work your lower abs in a manner similar to reverse curls. Slightly tilt your pelvis up, contract your lower abdominals, and slightly push your lower back flat. Hold for 8-10 seconds, then release. Repeat until reps are completed.

Exercise 5: Punch and Twist: Stan with your feet shoulder width apart, knees slightly bent. Bring your arms up to punching position. Twist to the left with the right hand punching toward the left corner of the room. Repeat the motion with the left hand punching toward the right corner of the room. 1 rep is a punch to each side. Do three sets of 5-10 reps.

Muscles Worked: Upper abs and Obliques

TIPS: Keep your body stationary when punching from side to side. Don't lean forward or backwards, stand straight and tall. Keep the movement small and controlled. Keep abdominal muscles contracted during the movements.

Everyday Version: While standing with your feet comfortably apart, knees bent bring your hands to your waist and twist slowly from side to side. 1 rep is a twist to each side. Repeat until reps are completed.

The other areas of concern identified by most people, are the buttocks (and hips) and thighs. Unfortunately for women, men have it much better in this part of the body. Heavier thighs and

buttocks are a gender factor than an age-related phenomenon. But, the good news for everyone is

the muscles of the lower body are the largest group in our bodies, which means they burn the most

calories (when toned or used).

Walking is by far the easiest, safest way to firm and tone the lower body. Biking, outside or inside on a stationary cycle is also an excellent toning as well as great cardiovascular exercise. The main goal with the lower body is the same as the rest of the body, *movement. Sitting itself doesn't necessarily determine where fat is deposited but a sedentary lifestyle in general does that. Your muscles would be far more toned if you were more active. Purposeful exercise can make up for the kind of sedentary lifestyle that puts on the pounds overall. But to see a real difference in your lower body, you will have to add resistance training to the mix. And remember,* the resistance used can be your own body weight. As with any exercise, there is a right and wrong way to go about working your lower body. Here are the 5 lower body exercise that I recommend for their simplicity and efficacy.

The 'KEEP IT MOVING" Lower Body Series:

Exercise 1: Lunges: Stand with your feet about 6 inches apart with toes facing forward. With your hands on hips, step forward with our left foot as far as possible, bending your right knee as you do. Lunge until your right knee almost touches the floor, and then slowly return to starting position. Do one set, and then repeat with the opposite leg. Do three sets of 5-10 reps.

Muscles Worked: Quadriceps (Front thighs), gluteals (buttocks)

TIPS: Keep your upper body from leaning forward by looking straight ahead. Don't let your knee go past your toes as you bend.

Everyday Version: Choose the stairs over elevators whenever possible. If there are stairs where you work, climb one flight for two weeks; increase the number of flights by 1 every 2 weeks. Or walk up and down the stairs in your home 3 to 5 times extra every day.

Exercise 2: Squats: Stand with your feet shoulder-width apart. Tighten your abdomen and stand straight. Lower yourself into a squatting position where your thighs are parallel to the ground. Return to starting position. Do three sets of 5-10 reps.

Muscles Worked: Quadriceps, gluteals

TIPS: Keep your knees in line with your feet as you squat. Don't drop your buttocks lower than your knees.

Everyday Version: Squat to pick up or lift objects. This movement is safer than bending and you will be less likely to injure your lower back.

Exercise 3: Standing Abductions: Holding onto a wall for balance, stand with your knees slightly bent, facing one side. Lift the outer leg to the side with foot flexed as far up as you can without moving your upper body. Return to starting position. Do one set, and then repeat on the opposite leg. Do three sets of 5-10 reps.

Muscle Worked: Gluteals and abductors (outer thighs)

TIPS: Use the muscles of the outer thigh and hip to lift the leg. Keep the supporting leg slightly bent. Keep your upper body still.

Everyday Version: While standing, contract your buttocks, hold for 6-10 seconds, and then release. Do for 1 to 3 minutes, 2-3 times a day.

Exercise 4: Front Knee Lifts: Stand with feet shoulder- width apart. Lift one leg to waist height, while supporting yourself on supporting leg. Return leg to starting position. Alternate to opposite leg for one repetition. Do three sets of 5-10 reps.

Muscles Worked: Quadriceps

TIPS: Keep upper body still. Don't swing the legs. Use the muscle to lift the leg and knee.

Everyday Version: Stand in place and lift each knee to waist level, alternating legs. Do for 1 to 5 minutes, 2-3 times a day.

Exercise 5: Rear Leg Lifts: Stand facing a wall for support. Extend one leg behind, bent at a 90 degree angle with your foot flexed. Lift knee and thigh until you feel the contraction in your buttocks. Return to staring position. Do one set, and then repeat on opposite leg. Do three sets of 5-10 reps.

Muscles Worked: Hamstrings (back of thighs), gluteals

TIPS: Use one slow, continuous, controlled motion throughout the exercise. Use your buttock and thigh, not momentum, to raise your leg.

Everyday Version: Spend 3 to 5 minutes going up and down a stepladder for 30 seconds at a time, with a15 second rest between intervals.

These are just a few easy, simple exercises to get you started and get your muscles used to being worked. Take your time and practice good form to keep safe from injury.

I also recommend stretching before and after any workout. Experts recommend that you stretch all your muscle groups, not just the trouble spots. All your muscles and tendons work together, so if you ignore one group, then you won't get maximum benefit from the others. Stretching should come fairly naturally. We raise our arms when we get out of bed; we wiggle our backs if we feel a muscle ache. All of these motions are really stretches.

Stretching doesn't take much time and you really don't need any equipment. If you are going to stretch on the floor, a towel will do nicely. If you've just stared working-out, its best to stretch each muscle group immediately after working those muscles. For example, if you are doing squats, stretch the gluteus immediately after the exercise. If you've been working out for awhile and are comfortable with your routine, feel free to do all your stretches at the end of your workout. The important thing is that you stretch. You can even stretch in front of the TV, there's no reason to be formal about it.

One last thought about the benefits of exercise. Exercise I both a stimulant and a tranquilizer. Believe it or not, exercise is also a great way to relax. Yes, I said relax. Exercise

relaxes you in several ways. Aerobic exercise releases natural chemicals, endorphins, that

automatically improve your mood and make you feel better. No matter how much or how little I

exercise, I always feel better afterward. Exercise also helps disperse adrenalin common in people who

are stressed out. A walk around the neighborhood or in a different environment can help you to relax

by getting away from whatever is bothering you, and let your mind wander. Getting out in the fresh air, looking at all the beauty that nature

provides is relaxing all by itself. And by the time you return from your walk, you probably won't even

remember what you were concerned about. Stretching helps relax tight muscles that may be holding

built up lactic acid that can make you feel stiff and sore. So now you know that you can use exercise

as a way to wind down as you let your body and mind recharge their energy levels.

Chapter 6

Food is Your Friend

Food is the fuel your body breaks down into the building blocks of life. Food sustains us and enables us to take on the challenges of everyday life. Despite the growing problem of obesity in this country, food is not the enemy. Short-term fad diets, diet pills, and quick fixes of every kind are the real enemies. Food is definitely your friend. There are no inherently "bad foods". You can develop a healthy relationship with food and enjoy every food that you desire, within moderation.

Good food is truly one of life's simple pleasures. Eating well and healthful does not have to be complicated or boring. Food is brilliantly colored fruits and vegetables, hearty grains, lean meats, rich dairy, and fresh fish captured from living rivers and oceans. Food is an enjoyable aspect of life that we should take pleasure in and appreciate. Food gives our bodies strength, helps to heal us when we are ill, and helps us to feel satisfied and comforted when we are hungry.

We are the most affluent country in the world, and we are the fattest. Forty percent of the population is twenty or more pounds overweight. How did so many people get so overweight? The answers are simple; we are eating too much and not exercising enough. The obvious solution is to eat less. But the problem of an overweight society comes from a combination of factors.

First, portion sizes have increased. We are eating more food. As a matter of fact if we go to a restaurant and we don't get a gigantic amount of food, we are not happy. Portion sizes have increased dramatically in the last 20 years. The average daily intake of adults rose by about 300 calories between 1985 and 2000. That means we have to work a lot harder to burn the extra calories that those larger portions add, and that's just not happening.

Secondly, we are eating more processed foods that have fewer nutrients. Over half the food available in America today is processed. We are also consuming a lot more added sugars hidden in carbonated drinks, fruit drinks, sports drinks, and processed foods. Research shows that between

1977 and 1997, the consumption of sugar-sweetened beverages, like soft drinks and fruit juices rose

by 61 percent. As a matter of fact, today many children get from 500 to 1000 calories a day from

these drinks alone. Evidence suggests that drinking calorie-laden beverages may not even make you feel full. This can lead you to drink more than you need, adding even more insidious calories to your diet.

We also eat out more than ever before. Most of us grew up only eating out on "special occasions". But with the advent of the two working parent scenario, lack of time and outright convenience has led many working couples to feed their children and themselves "the quickest meal possible". The danger is that many types of food eaten away from home, especially fast food and many take-home grocery items are high in saturated fat, sodium, cholesterol, and added sugars. So what seems to be a harmless, good, and easy solution to the food and time crunch actually isn't good at all. These foods can also be low in fiber, vitamins and minerals. So we wind up eating a bunch of "empty food". Not only that, but because we have paid for "eating out", we feel compelled to eat everything that we are served, so we wind up eating a lot more.

The third factor that has contributed to America's overweight problem is we are less active as a nation. Current estimates indicate that over half of the adults in the United States do not engage in *any regular physical activity. As more and more children, as well as adults, spend more time in front of televisions, video games, and computers, more are likely to put on pounds. Our increasingly sedentary lifestyles are putting us at risk for serious health problems including cardiovascular disease, type II diabetes, osteoporosis, depression, and colon cancer.*

American children are less active too, and heavier than in any other time in history. They are now at risk for conditions that usually don't develop until adulthood. Do you know the most important predictor of childhood obesity is? It is obese parents. Obesity actually begins in the cradle. Sadly, many American mothers have misconceptions about feeding their children that increases that their children will become obese. Many health experts believe that after the age of five, the situation really boils down to this: Children and teens eat too much and exercise too little. When people don't

understand the mechanism of metabolism, they mistakenly shut down their metabolism by *not eating,*

which in turn triggers the body to store fat, which is the last thing they are trying to accomplish!

Instead of watching our weight, we need to get really smart about the most effective ways to burn off

excess fat automatically and continually by using our body's natural "engine" as an ally and a potent

weapon against "aging weight gain".   That natural engine is our metabolism and learning to maximize

its efficiency is key to maintaining a healthy weight. To get your metabolic engine going, you have to

"stoke the furnace" with food.

Most people don't understand that when you finally break your overnight or midday fast and have a meal, you are more likely to overeat and make poor food choices. And, the longer you make your body wait between meals, the less efficient it becomes at burning fat, and the more muscle tissue you sacrifice to glucose production. So if you skip breakfast and make your body wait until lunch to get any nutrition, *you are actually teaching your body to slow down metabolism and store fat. Muscle cells, unlike fat cells, are active; they actually work. Remember, the mitochondria are like little energy plants and are responsible for burning many of the calories we take in each day. So when you lose muscle, you lose some of your body's ability to burn calories. When the body uses up muscle tissue to compensate for the "starvation" of not eating, it accomplishes two things at once. It gets extra energy but also slows down your metabolism in the process. As you now know, when it comes to building a firm body, muscle breakdown is the virtual kiss-of death.*

A fundamental key to healthful body weight is eating in order to maintain or lose weight. For most people, breakfast is the first meal of the day after a stretch of 8 to 12 hours with little or no food. Starting off any "machine" with the right kind of fuel is important to keep it functioning properly, and recent research has linked an amazing array of health and wellness benefits to the regular consumption of breakfast.

Many people mistakenly shut down their metabolism by not eating. By using our metabolism as a natural "engine", when we give it fuel it burns calories. When our metabolism slows or stops due to lack of food, our body is signaled to store fat. To get the metabolic engine burning, you have to "stoke" the furnace with food.

The longer the body waits between meals, the less efficient it becomes at burning fat. If you skip breakfast and wait until lunch to break the overnight fast, you are teaching your body to slow down metabolism and store fat. This occurrence is known as the starvation response. It is an automatic, innate physiological response to the lack of food.

Breakfast breaks the 8 to 12 hour fast that occurs from the last meal of the day until the first meal of the new day. What we forget is that while we are asleep, our brain and body are still at work. Muscles rebuild themselves, food is digested, and heart and lungs continue to function. The brain busy processing data collected throughout the day, oversees the entire complex operation, burning up a huge amount of fuel in the form of glucose. So when you get out of bed in the morning, your brain and body at in a huge calorie deficit.

If it takes all your mental firepower just to get coffee going in the morning, then you are probably n ot interested in the optimal nutritional breakdown of your morning meal. The most important action at this point, is to eat something. Colorful, unprocessed foods are the best choice. The rest of the breakfast should contain a combination of lean protein and complex carbohydrates, which are slowly digested and help to maintain a steady blood sugar. Experiment with different meals based on what you like to eat. For example, if you are a 'sweets' person try whole –grain French toast (the egg is the protein) with strawberries and maple syrup; or a smoothie with blueberries, orange juice and a scoop of protein powder. If you prefer a more savory breakfast try: A whole-wheat tortilla with scrambled egg black beans, and sliced avocado or sliced turkey breast on whole wheat toast, with lettuce, tomato and cucumber. And finally, if you are just not a person try; a banana and raw almonds, or a ready-made protein drink.

When eaten within an hour of waking, a healthy meal brings your blood sugar back check, fires up your metabolism; kick starts your cognitive processes, and regulates your mood. Both adults and children who eat breakfast tend to perform better at certain types of tasks, such as memory recall, visual perception, spatial analysis, problem solving, and basic math. Adults who start their day with a healthy breakfast tend to have healthier body weight, better hunger regulation throughout the day and make better food choices. Kids who eat a healthy breakfast tend to have higher standardized test scores, higher levels of motivation and academic performance, fewer health complaints during the day, and are at a lower risk for developing obesity.

On the other side of the issue, if you make a habit of skipping your morning meal, you could be setting yourself up for a lot of problems throughout the day. To not refuel by eating breakfast is an invitation to throw your body into distress. So it is counterproductive not to eat breakfast. Studies have consistently shown that skipping breakfast keeps the body in a fasting mode and is a stressful state for the body. To compensate for the lack of fuel, people generally eat larger, heavier meals later in the day and often into the night to make up for the lack of an early morning meal. Breakfast deprived adults tend to have higher LDL ,("bad") cholesterol, higher levels of insulin resistance and may be at greater risk of heart disease. Making breakfast an essential part of your daily routine will yield major health benefits and ensure better performance and more efficient function throughout the day.

When you eat a meal the body has to break down the food, then absorb and process the nutrients for distribution throughout your system. This process burns energy. This phenomenon is known as the thermogenic effect of a meal and is most pronounced during the first 90 minutes after a meal. The more frequently you eat a small meal or snack, the more thermogenic activity is generated by the body and the more calories are burned as a result of eating. The remaining calories are either used to fuel the body's functions or stored as fat. In other words, a person who eats five 300 calorie meals throughout the day will have a faster metabolism and burn more calories between meals than a person who eats three 500 calorie meals instead.

Also known as the thermic effect of food, dietary thermogenesis, or diet-induced thermogenesis, DIT, is the process of energy production in the body caused directly by the metabolizing of food consumed. Dietary thermogenesis is influenced by factors relating to the composition of the food and the physical state of the individual. A 2004 analysis published in " Nutrition and Metabolism" of research on dietary thermogenesis found that in an energy-balanced state, a mixed diet of proteins, fats and carbohydrates produced an energy expenditure from dietary thermogenesis that constituted 5 to 15 percent of total daily energy expenditure.

Factors relating to the food you eat could influence their associated rate of dietary thermogenesis, in particular their energy content, or calories, and macronutrient composition. A 2008 study reported in "Metabolism" found that eating protein produces greater dietary thermogenesis than eating fat. The dietary thermogenic value of carbohydrates falls somewhere between protein and fat.

The 2011 study further suggested that a low rate of dietary thermogenesis following frequent or recurring fat consumption could be a factor in obesity.

The clear winner when it comes to food that burns the most calories in the digestion process is protein. Protein has often been called muscle food. The 22 amino acids in protein are used primarily not for fuel but to form the structural components of muscle. In fact, the amino acids in protein are used to build and repair most dynamic body systems, including all the enzymes

necessary for fat metabolism. Without adequate protein our muscles
could not repair and grow from exercise, nor could they keep up with day-to-day maintenance. Protein is the best nutrient
for producing the sensation of feeling full and also helps build muscle and keeps your metabolism cranked up, giving you
more energy as you burn more calories. To get the maximum benefit from protein you need to know which foods are best
and how to incorporate those foods into your diet at regular intervals.

Protein is broken down by the digestive system into long chains of amino acids which are
released into the bloodstream. The body uses the amino acids to make new proteins for tissue
building and to create enzymes, hormones, hemoglobin and other functional proteins. Our bodies are
able to make some amino acids, but the rest come from food. The best way to get enough of these
essential amino acids is by choosing high quality protein sources.

Unlike fats and carbohydrates, proteins are not stored. The protein induced thermogenesis
requires the body to burn calories just to metabolize the protein ingested during a meal. An optimal
protein intake instantly increases fat burning. In fact, a protein rich meal or snack can burn 40
percent more calories than a high carbohydrate alternative.

Recent research has shown that high-protein, moderate-carbohydrate, lower-fat meals produce a g
reater sense of long lasting fullness than high fat meals. The chief reason for this phenomenon is
that protein breaks down more slowly than fat and even more slowly than carbohydrates. Since
protein satisfies the feeling of hunger well and intensifies calorie expenditure, it is front and center on
the list of foods that will help you get to and maintain your desired weight which in turn will enhance
your level of fitness.

Protein triggers the production of glucagon, the hormone that enables the body to use fat as fuel
instead of storing it. Glucagon is essential for building new muscle tissue, as well as for boosting

energy. According to studies by a research scientist at MIT, protein tends to change neurotransmitter balance in favor of alertness which indicates an active metabolism

Researchers have also discovered that natural protein supports the production and secretion of human growth hormone (HGH). Enhanced production of HGH appears to enhance fat-burning and energy production in both men and women. Consuming protein rich food or drink after exercise may elevate the secretion of HGH. There are many great sources of protein and other "fitness friendly" foods that are readily available, of moderate to low cost, and easy to incorporate into your diet.

The way we eat is as important as what we eat. Making each eating experience meaningful and satisfying, creating an aesthetically pleasing setting for meals, eating from nice dinnerware with corresponding glassware and silverware, helps us truly enjoy the experience. Emphasize quality over quantity, eating slowly, and savoring the unique texture and flavor of each food. Most importantly, learn to stop eating when satisfied, not full. Learning that less can be more and discovering how one can eat everything in moderation are keys. Highlight the value of fresh seasonal foods and use of fruits and vegetables in abundance as well as fresh herbs and spices to enhance the taste of food without extra calories. Remember the importance of breakfast, as well as eating three meals a day as a way to keep the metabolism functioning at an efficient and steady rate. Prepare as much food as possible at home to control what and how much you are eating. Focus on a wide variety of foods to prevent boredom. Consume an abundant array of fruits and vegetables to provide many health benefits. Do not deprive yourself of any food, so all foods are to be enjoyed without guilt. Increase your awareness of portion size and enjoy the act of eating. Do not judge your successes by obsessive attention to calories, carbohydrates, proteins, fats, or other chemical structures. You would be bored to death thinking about such things, especially when applying it to a part of life that should be considered sacred; food and its enjoyment.

Here are a few healthful suggestions that you may want to consider as you adjust your eating style:

Wet Your Whistle. You have heard this from childhood; drink 8 glasses of water every day. As it turns out, that was very sage advice. I have discovered important facts that may make you more inclined to reach for another glass of water.

We all know that drinking water just before a meal helps make you feel full and encourages you to eat less. Additionally, water my help burn calories. According to a study done in Germany in 2003, healthy normal weight volunteers were given 2 cups of water and within 10 minutes their metabolisms had begun to increase. After 30 to 40 minutes, their metabolisms had increased by an average of 30 percent. Healthy, normal weight volunteers were given two cups of water to drink, and within 10 minutes, their metabolic rate had begun to rev up.   The researchers who conducted this study estimated that 40 percent of this increase was due to the heating of the water from room temperature to body temperature while the remainder was attributed to an increase in fat and carbohydrate burning stimulated by the sympathetic nervous system. These findings support that the recommended eight glasses of water per day will burn off a very significant additional 100 calories on the days that you drink 8 glasses.

In addition, there may be some added advantage to drinking ice-cold water. When you drink ice water, your body temperature falls, and in order to return it to normal, your body has to generate energy by burning calories. It takes 80 calories to heat two quarts of water from 32 degrees (freezing) to the normal temperature of 98.6 degrees. So just by drinking eight 8 ounces glasses of ice water each day, you could potentially burn 160 calories without even trying. Since we have to drink water to survive anyway, this little known benefit of drinking cold water is worth a try whether you are trying to lose weight or just quench your thirst.

The researchers who conducted this study estimated that 40 percent of this increase was due the body's effort to heat the ingested water to body temperature. These findings support the recommended 8 glasses of water per day could potentially help burn an additional 100 calories on the days you consume all 8 glasses.

Shop for seafood. **Fish seems to be particularly effective at turning up the body's thermostat. Several studies have shown that people who eat lots of seafood have lower levels leptin, a hormone that beefs up appetite and fat storage, and are less likely to be overweight. It turns out that this may be because of the omega-3 fatty acids that are especially abundant in mackerel, sardines, tuna, and other cold-water, fatty fish. Wild salmon is especially recommended because not only is it high in protein, it also contains an abundance of omega-3**

and omega-6 fatty acids. These "good" fats are essential for energy production and fat loss. When these fats replace other fats in animal diets, there is a decreased weight gain and accumulation of fat in the abdominal area, along with improved metabolism of fats and glucose

The fish doesn't have to be fancy or expensive, canned tuna and salmon are great choices for high quality protein. Most other fish and seafood enhance the efficiency of the hormone lep tin, which also helps to reduce fat cell size and enhances fat loss. Fish oil capsules are also an option for those who do not like to eat fish and they provide omega-3 fatty acids.

Eat Skinless Chicken and Turkey. I'm sure that you already eat a lot of chicken, as most of us

do. As a matter of fact, some weeks I'm sure I'm about ready to sprout wings and fly as a

result of all of the chicken I eat. But I have recently discovered several different Turkey

products that I really enjoy. For example, I use ground Turkey for tacos,

Eat an egg. Eggs are an excellent source of protein and they contain no saturated fat. Eggs are portable, readily available, easy to cook, and versatile. Moderation is the key with egg consumption. Servings should be limited to 2-3 times per week.

Grab a' Cup of Joe. Over 18,000 studies have looked at coffee use in the past few decades.   C offee has recently been found to have a number of health benefits. It enhances cognitive performance, quickens reaction time, and promotes alertness and sustained attention. It restores fading energy, can stop migraine headaches, boost mood, relieve symptoms of asthma and even prevent cavities. It improves endurance so much that Olympic athletes can be disqualified for using high doses of caffeine. In addition, coffee is a good source of antioxidants. As a matter of fact, a 2005 study revealed Americans get more antioxidants from coffee than from any other source. In recent decades many studies have been done examining coffee's impact on health. And for the most part, their results have been as pleasing as the first sip of freshly brewed coffee. Overall, the research conducted at Vanderbilt University's Institute for Coffee Studies shows that coffee is far more healthful than harmful.

Nibble On Nuts. Recently nuts have come into popularity compact source of protein and fiber. As a new nutritional era emerges that moves beyond macronutrients like fat and protein into the world of phytonutrients, nutritionists are rediscovering the power of nuts. People who eat nuts regularly can enjoy a significant reduction in their risk of developing coronary artery disease. They will also reduce their risk of diabetes, cancer, and a host of chronic ailments.

All nuts and significant are significant contributors to good health. There are hundreds of nuts to consider but there are 4 that top the nutrition list. Walnuts top the category of nuts as a super food. They are one of the few rich sources of plant-derived omega-3 fatty acids. They are rich in plant sterols which can play a significant role in lowering serum cholesterol levels. Walnuts are also rich in arginine, which is an essential amino acid. Arginine helps to keep the inside of   blood vessels smooth while promoting vessel flexibility thus increasing blood flow while reducing blood pressure. They are also a good source of fiber and protein. Walnuts also provide magnesium, copper, folate, vitamin E, and they are the nut with the highest antioxidant activity.

Peanuts are America's favorite nuts, even though they are not really nuts at all. Peanuts are legumes which makes them closely related to beans. They are considered nuts because of their similar nutritional profile. Peanuts make up two-thirds of the nation's nut consumption and rank third in snack food sales. One ounce, (48 nuts) provides 15 percent of the daily requirement for Vitamin E, 2.5 grams of fiber plus calcium, copper, zinc, niacin, folate, iron, and magnesium, along with 7 grams of protein.

Almonds are the best nut source of vitamin E and a powerful plant source of protein. One quarter cup of almond contains 7.6 grams of protein, more than a large egg which only contains 6 grams. Almonds also contain riboflavin, iron, potassium, magnesium, and fiber. Almonds are also an excellent source of the B vitamin biotin, an essential element needed for the metabolism of both sugar and fat. One-quarter cup of almonds provides 75 percent of the body's daily requirement of this nutrient, which promotes skin health and energy. Almonds are also rich in arginine, a natural vasodilator which promotes increased blood flow by relaxing blood vessel walls.

Pistachios are one of the oldest edible nuts on earth. In China they are known as the happy nut because of their characteristic half-opened shell. A one-ounce serving is equal to 47 nuts. Pistachios are loaded with fiber; more than contained in a half-cup of broccoli or spinach. Pistachios are also rich in potassium, thiamine, and B6of cancers.. Like all nuts, pistachios are particularly rich in the phytonutrients associated with reducing cholesterol and protecting against a variety of cancers.

A large body of evidence now conclusively demonstrates that nut consumption correlates with reduced coronary artery disease. To date, at least five large epidemiological studies have demonstrated that frequent consumption of nuts decrease the risk of coronary artery disease. In each of these studies when an average of 5 servings of nuts were consumed per week, the lower the risk. Even when the results were adjusted for other factors such as age, race, and lifestyle variables, the conclusions were the same. Overall, people who ate nuts five times or more a week had a 15 to 51 percent reduction in coronary artery disease. Even people who ate nuts just once a month had some reduction.

One of the main contributors th heart health in nuts, particularly in walnuts, is the omega-3 fatty acids. It is widely known that omega-3 fatty acids work in various ways to help guarantee a healthy heart and circulatory system. Like aspirin, omega-3s "thin" the blood, helping it to flow freely while preventing clots from forming and adhering to vessel walls. Omega-3s also act as an anti-inflammatory by preventing the blood vessels from becoming inflamed, thereby reducing the amount of blood that flows through the vessel. Lowered blood pressure is an additional benefit of the omega-3s which is another way of decreasing the risk of cardiovascular disease.

While some types of nuts are higher in fat, most contain unsaturated fats that help reduce bad LDL cholesterol. According to a study from Purdue University, almonds appear to aid weight loss. Although the mechanism is unclear, researchers speculate that the protein in nuts may help burn more calories during the digestive process. Nuts are high in fat, so portion size is important.

Befriend Beans. Beans are a virtual wonder food because they are one of the healthiest and most economical sources of protein available. In addition beans are delicious source of vitamin-rich, low-fat, inexpensive, source of fiber, and are among the most humble sources of nutritional versatility. Beans are rich in soluble fiber which helps to balance blood sugar. Beans also help

prevent insulin resistance that can lead to fat gain. But the full
power of beans to lower cholesterol; combat heart disease; stabilize blood sugar; reduce
obesity; relieve constipation, diverticular disease, and lessen the risk for cancer make this
ancient food an extraordinary and important addition to any meal plan.
Toss In Tomatoes: In addition to being cancer-protective, there is significant evidence that
tomatoes also play a role in reducing the risk for cardiovascular disease. The antioxidant
function of lycopene, combined with the other powerful antioxidants in tomatoes such as
Vitamin C and beta-carotene work in the body to neutralize free radicals that could otherwise damage
cells and cell membranes. This preservation of cells and their membranes reduces the potential for
the progression and severity of atherosclerosis (clogged arteries). In one study, German scientists com
pared lycopene levels in the tissues of men who had suffered heart attacks with those men who had
not. The men who had suffered attacks had lower lycopene levels than those who had not.

Lycopene, a member of the carotenoid family and a pigment that contributes to the red color of
tomatoes, is a major contributor to their health-promoting power. Lycopene has demonstrated a range
of distinct and unique biological properties that have intrigued scientists and prompted further study of
this substance. Some researchers believe that lycopene could be as powerful an antioxidant as beta-
carotene.

Attention on lycopene began in the 1980s when studies started to reveal that people who ate large
amounts of tomatoes were far less likely to die from all forms of cancer compared to those who ate
little or no tomatoes. Many other studies have verified the positive findings about the effect of eating
tomatoes. Lycopene also plays an important role in the antioxidant network in the skin. Dietary lycope
ne, by itself or in combination with other nutrients, can raise the sun protection factor (SPF) of skin. In
other words by eating tomatoes, especially cooked or processed, you can enhance your skin's ability
to protect itself from the damaging rays of the sun acting as an internal sun block.

Lycopene is rare in foods and tomatoes are only one of a few that are rich in this powerful
antioxidant. Ketchup, tomato juice, and pizza sauce account for 80 percent of the total intake of
Americans. Red watermelon is another excellent source of lycopene. A very concentrated,
bioavailable source of the nutrient watermelon may be even richer in lycopene than tomatoes.
Spice up your Life. All spices have health benefits. Culinary spices do more than just turn up
the flavor of foods they also serve up unique health benefits including aiding, your fat burning
mechanisms. All spices, which are derived from bark, seeds, or fruit help to detoxify the body.
They are also potent anti-inflammatories. They are part of your environmental shield, as they
rev up Phase 2 enzymes that block cancer, and help further reduce cancer risk by stimulating

apoptosis, or programmed cell death. Your body has the ability to **identify unhealthy cells; it first tries to help sick cells, and if they don't respond it kills them off When programmed cell death does not work properly, the cells that should be eliminated linger and become mutated as in cancer and leukemia.**

These fat-burning catalysts include cayenne, black pepper, cinnamon, and ginger. While the effects of these spices are mild, they do increase thermogenesis.

Remember when you broke out into a sweat after eating hot peppers? Peppers contain a compound called *capsaicin, which is responsible for the heat and makes cayenne the best of the thermogenic spices. In addition to boosting metabolism, capsaicin has also been shown to suppress appetite. When researchers added red pepper powder to tomato juice or gave capsaicin capsules to study volunteers 30 minutes before meals, they reported feeling fullers sooner and ate less at meal time.*

Black pepper is the most popular spice in the United States and may also be an ally in your battle against weight gain. A substance in black pepper called piperine may help block the formation of new fat cells, according to a recent study on mice from the *Journal of Agricultural and Food Chemistry.*

If you've hit the gym or the yard a little too hard recently, a sprinkle of cinnamon may help you recover faster. *Women who ate about 1 ½ teaspoons of cinnamon everyday for six weeks experienced a decrease in muscle soreness brought on by exercise according to research from the International Journal Of Preventive Medicine.*

Although you know ginger best as a stomach soother, it may also help you feel fuller and even burn more calories. When overweight men ate breakfast with ginger tea, they felt more satisfied and ate less throughout the day than men who were given the same breakfast with just hot water, says *Metabolism. Plus the men who drank ginger tea burned about 40 calories just digesting their meal.*

Additional health benefits associated with other spices include:

- Anise for its anti-inflammatory properties and because it promotes pulmonary health.
- Caraway because it promotes digestive health and has antimicrobial action.
- Clove for its anti-cancer, anti-inflammatory properties.
- Cumin for its detoxification properties.
- Fennel because it promotes digestive health.
- Marjoram because helps atopic skin diseases and may help protect against Alzheimer's.
- Nutmeg for its anti-inflammatory and anticancer properties.
- Oregano for its antioxidant, antifungal, antibacterial, and lung protection properties.
- Rosemary for its antioxidant, anti-inflammatory, detoxification properties.
- Sage for its antioxidant properties.

- Thyme for its anti-cancer properties.
- Turmeric for its cancer-fighting and Alzheimer's prevention properties.

Don't Forget Dairy . There is more and more evidence suggesting that people who consume low-fat dairy products on a regular basis are less likely to be overweight. Besides their protein content, dairy products are the best dietary sources of calcium which has been town to elevate metabolism, prevent fat storage and help the body burn existing fat.

Yogurt is a great source of readily digestible protein. In fact, yogurt delivers twice the protein of milk because it is usually thickened with non fat milk solids, increasing its protein content. Some people, especially the elderly don't consume enough protein or calcium. Studies have shown there is a positive correlation between protein intake and bone-mineral density of older women and men when they are supplemented with calcium.

Optimal bone health and prevention of osteoporosis require both sufficient calcium and protein intake. Yogurt with its easily digestible protein and calcium is a convenient way to fulfill both requirements. Low fat yogurt is an excellent dairy source that comes in a variety of flavors and textures, with Greek yogurt having the additional benefit of extra protein in each serving.

One of my favorite breakfasts is a quick and easy on-the-go favorite. I take a carton of non-fat, Greek yogurt and top it with a handful of dried, mixed berries, a few walnut pieces, and a drizzle of honey. It is a delicious, nutritious and portable meal.

There is another group of foods that are extremely beneficial for our health. This group is known as "functional "foods. Although you may not be familiar with this term, you have probably been eating them all along. Functional foods do more than meet your minimum daily requirements of nutrients. They also play a role in reducing the risk of disease and the promotion of good health.

While all foods are function as a source of nutrition, functional foods contain health-promoting ingredients that benefit the body. This category of food includes whole foods as well as fortified, enriched, and enhanced foods. Most of us have been eating rudimentary types of functional foods for years in the form of vitamin fortified cereals, iron-enriched breads; and vitamin A and D fortified milk.

At that time, fortification was done to prevent nutritional deficiencies that could result in rickets, scurvy, and other diseases of malnutrition.

The concept of functional foods is not new, although dramatic advances have been made recently. Swiss pharmacist Henri Nestle' concocted one of the world's first functional foods on 1867. He paved the way for bottle feeding by inventing baby formula. Nestle's baby-food-in a bottle idea gave millions of infants who would have died without their mother's milk a second chance at life. Early in the 1900s, food manufacturers in the United States began adding iodine to salt to prevent goiters (an enlargement of the thyroid gland), representing one of the first attempts at creating a functional component through fortification. Today researchers have identified hundreds of compounds with functional qualities, and they continue to make new discoveries about the complex benefits of phytochemicals (plant chemicals) in foods. Phytochemicals are found in many foods and have been noted to provide many benefits beyond basic nutrition. Some studies have even noted that certain types of tea and chocolate have beneficial health benefits.

Research has shown that many fruit, vegetables, grains, fish, and dairy and meat products contains several natural components that deliver benefits beyond basic nutrition, such as lycopene in tomatoes, omega-3 fatty acids in salmon, and saponins in soybeans. Other foods get a boost during processing with added nutrients or other ingredients. This is true of orange juice fortified with calcium, cereals with added vitamins or minerals and flour with added folic acid. In fact, more foods are being fortified with nutrients as researchers uncover evidence about the nutrients' role in health and disease-risk reduction. The scientific community has just begun to understand the interactions between nutritional components and the human body. However there is already a large body of scientific evidence that shows eating functional foods on a regular basis as part of a varied diet can help reduce the risk or decrease the severity of many health concerns related to aging. As the knowledge about functional food grows, so does the interest in eating functional food for the potential health benefits. Here is a list of the top 10 functional foods. Look at the list and determine which ones, if included in your eating plan, could help keep you healthy. You will not be familiar, or en like some of the foods listed below. But don't let that stop you from trying to find one or two you can add to your diet. Try new fruits and vegetables, surprise yourself.

1. SOY: Soy is good food and can be added to your diet in a number of ways. Tofu, edemame (soybeans), soy milk, and soy flour are just a few sources.

2.   TOMATOES: Tomatoes offer vitamin C and a lot more.   They are rich in carotenoids, including lycopene, a relative of beta-carotene. An interesting fact just recently discovered is cooked and processed tomatoes have 10 times the lycopene, ounce for ounce.

3. NUTS: Nuts have always been valued for their protein, vitamins, and minerals. They are also rich in monosaturated fats like the kind found in olive oil, fiber, vitamin E, Folic acid and other B vitamins.

4. GARLIC: The garlic family, including the onion-family members such as chives, shallots, leeks, and scallions (green onions), contains allylic sulfides and other compounds that may reduce the risk of cancerous tumors. Benefits to the heart, blood pressure, and suppression of LDL (bad cholesterol) have also been demonstrated in some studies.

5. FISH: Fatty fish such as salmon, tuna, mackerel and sardines contain large amounts of omega-3 fatty acids that are known to reduce the risk of heart disease.

6. OATS & GRAINS: Oats, oat bran, and whole-oat products contain the soluble fiber beta-glucan, which aids in decreasing blood cholesterol levels by binding with bile acids in the intestine, helping to carry cholesterol out of the body. Wheat germ, brown rice, corn bran, oatmeal and whole wheat breads are good sources of insoluble fiber which act like a broom in the body, sweeping away the waste.

7. COLORED FRUITS & VEGETABLES: Deeply colored fruits and vegetables tend to have the most vitamins and minerals. Also the pigments have high antioxidant potential and may help protect against some diseases.

8. TEA: Most teas, though not herb teas, contain a variety of potentially beneficial phyto- chemicals that may reduce the risk of many cancers. Tea has an abundance of flavonoids called catechins,

which are a type of antioxidant.

9. PURPLE GRAPES: The purple grapes used to make red wine and purple grape juice have phytochemicals called polyphenolic compounds that support healthy heart function, help reduce plaque buildup in the arteries and help prevent LDL (bad cholesterol) from attaching to artery walls.

10.   CHOCOLATE: Chocolate contains large amounts of catechins, the
same compounds found in tea. One ounce of chocolate has as much beneficial catechins as one cup
of brewed black tea.

While the benefits of any food depend on a person's overall diet, the evidence that certain
foods provide specific health benefits and reduce the risk of certain diseases is rooted in scientific fact.
The most effective way to reap the health benefits from any type of food is to eat a variety
emphasizing fruits, vegetables, and foods that provide added health benefits. And while there are no
magic foods that can ever prevent us from contracting disease or cure disease, when we choose
healthier foods we are choosing to maintain our bodies at an optimal level.

Research has discovered that many fruit, vegetable, grains, meat, fish, and dairy products
contain several natural components that deliver benefits beyond basic nutrition. Phytochemicals, also
known as phytonutrients, are naturally occurring plant compounds that work with the body to fight
disease and boost health. Phytochemicals are very biologically active. They include antioxidants and
other compounds that modify toxins and carcinogens.

Thousands of Phytochemicals are found everywhere in the plant world, where they often function
as natural defenses against biological hazards. Phytochemicals give plants their color, flavor, and
natural disease resistance. Tomatoes are estimated to contain over 10,000 phytochemicals.
According to research, the best way to get the benefits from phytochemicals is by eating a variety of
foods.

Carotenoids are the most common Phytochemicals. They are responsible for the orange, red, and
yellow pigments found in fruits and vegetables. The most commonly named of the family are alpha-
carotene, beta-carotene, and lycopene. These Carotenoids are found in carrots, tomatoes, pumpkins,
watermelon, and broccoli just to name a few.

A federally funded study of 14,000 men and women tracked their eating patterns for 10 years
found the subjects who ate more cruciferous and leafy vegetables in their 60's had a lower rate of
decline on learning and memory tests. The more of these vegetables they ate, the better they

performed.

Vegetables and fruits are packed with antioxidants and other essential vitamins and minerals. Both groups are low in calories and full of fiber. Antioxidants help the body neutralize harmful free radicals and are involved in the process that helps the body and brain make energy. Eating a variety of fruits and vegetables will maximize your antioxidant intake. The American Heart Association recommends the goal of 5 servings of fruits and vegetables each day. Five servings sounds excessive but it really isn't and it's easy to do. Here is an example of this daily recommendation: 6oz of orange juice, 1 cup of leafy greens, ½ cup red tomatoes, ¼ cup yellow bell pepper, and ½ cup blueberries. In addition to the vitamins provided, it is also a visual rainbow of nutritious foods. The colors represented in foods are indicators of nutritional value and different colors mean different vitamins and minerals.

RED: Red-hued fruits and vegetables offer the important antioxidant lycopene. As previously mentioned, lycopene is antioxidant that is associated with many health benefits. Lycopene is the most strongly concentrated in the tomato.

ORANGE: Beta-carotene is the nutrient

Phytochemicals, also known as phytonutrients, are naturally occurring plant compounds that work with the body to fight disease and enhance health. They include antioxidants and other compounds that modify toxins and carcinogens. Thousands of phytochemicals are found in the plant world, where they of function as natural defenses against biological hazards. Phytochemicals give plants their color, flavor, and natural disease resistance. Phytochemicals react biochemically to one another w ithin the plant.

The best way to be satisfied is to eat foods with a variety of flavors, colors, and textures. Think of baby carrots, tossed salad with mixed greens and chopped yellow and red peppers. Vegetables are naturally high in fiber which is also a big part of healthful eating. Fiber is not sexy, but it can help you fit into the clothes that you can no longer wear. High-fiber foods are filling and they prevent you from overeating. Fiber-rich foods take up more space in your stomach, so you feel satisfied longer. Fiber is found in plant cell walls and cannot be digested by the human body. Fiber has no calories and is not broken down like other foods. It moves through your digestive system, virtually intact, so it provides calorie-free filler giving you a feeling of fullness.

The underlying cause for any weight problem is eating the wrong *amounts of food. Most people just plain eat too much, an average of 250 calories a day more than w 25 years ago. There are many reasons for the larger portion sizes of today, but businesses are responding to consumer demand. Americans simply want and consume the larger portion sizes.*

There really are no best or worst foods; only overall ways of eating that can be best or worst for you. You don't have to give up anything other than your old attitudes about food. You need to enjoy a variety of foods, not too much or too little of any one food. Cultivating a new food attitude means making better food decisions, not relying on willpower to avoid temptation. It's easier to stick to a healthful eating plan when you include some favorites. Plan your meals, shop from a list and go to the store on a full stomach. If you refrigerator is full of vegetables, fruits, protein and dairy products you have shopped wisely and your resolve to get and stay healthy will most likely remain strong.

Make yourself fully accountable for your eating choices; consciously decide what you put into your mouth. Let go of the all-or-nothing dieting mentality and gain some peace of mind. Nothing in life is black or white; everything is on a continuum of gray. Just because you ate more than you should at one meal doesn't translate to dietary disaster. Don't make one mistake the excuse for giving up on your decision to be aware of what you eat. To err is human. Accept responsibility for your food choices and realize you can increase your daily caloric intake when are working out on a regular basis.

If you plan what you are going to eat before going out to dinner, or to a party you are already one step ahead of the game. If you choose to treat yourself to your favorite indulgence, go ahead. Every indulgence doesn't have to turn into a binge. Have a small portion of decadence and really enjoy it. Never let yourself be at the mercy of food or the situation. Value yourself and let motivation for change come from within. You may be pleasantly surprised that mindful, food-friendly eating is a springboard for other positive changes in your life. If you are going to maintain a healthy weight in a lasting way, you need to understand the power of *good food*. *High quality protein, fresh vegetables, and fresh fruit fall under the category of good food. Good food actually balances your system and promotes health, whereas bad food creates unbalance and instability. When you take in bad food, your body suffers and in the same way, when you eat good food your body thrives. Consuming good food empowers you in a number of ways. Good food increases your energy level while decreasing your chances of developing illnesses. Eating well can also contribute to an overall youthful appearance and slow the aging process. Besides all that, eating healthy food facilitates weight loss because when you eat the right kinds of food, you feel fuller on fewer calories. When eating properly, you can eat more for less. When you eat good food, the calories are lower, but your body doesn't go into starvation mode. Eventually, your body adapts to the change in food and you will experience fewer cravings for unhealthy food.*

Here are a few simple suggestions to help get you started on food mastery. Slowly adopt these simple guidelines most for most days and you will manage to keep yourself at a trim, healthy weight. Here is a list of some foods I recommend for a beneficial, easy style of

eating. Try some of the ideas for a week and not only will you have lost weight,
you will also feel more energetic, less sluggish, and ready to live.

First and foremost, get rid of most of the "white" foods that you consume in your diet. All of
the bread, potatoes, white sugar, pasta, etc. Keep in mind that most of the foods that are high in
sugar are also high in calories and devoid of nutritional value. Food high in carbohydrates cause
spikes and valleys in blood sugar which make s it very difficult to manage your energy, and your
hunger. These foods taste good and satisfying while we are eating them, but they wreak havoc on our
bodies and can contribute to losing control. Now I'm not suggesting that all carbohydrates are bad.
That would be a ridiculous suggestion that is just not true. Carbohydrates contain essential nutrients
and many of our most healthful foods such as vegetables and fruits are composed primarily of
carbohydrates. But the difference between the carbohydrates in simple sugars and the
carbohydrates in fruits and vegetables is huge. What I am suggesting is that you consider the nutritive
value of any carbohydrate that you decide to eat.

The reason for decreasing the amount of white foods is that they are the lowest in
nutritional value and do the most damage to your body in terms of blood sugar and empty calories.
Most vegetables, legumes, and fruit promote slow sustained release of blood sugar. Starchy
carbohydrates rapidly drive up blood sugar. And all those low-fat, refined grain products that have
become a major part of our diet send sugar and insulin levels flying. A chain of detrimental events is
initiated inside your body when you feed it the wrong foods. Here is a synopsis of the carbohydrate-
insulin problem in a nut shell:

When you eat too much of the wrong kinds of carbohydrate it is quickly digested and
absorbed, and you get a huge rise in your blood sugar. This triggers a correspondingly large release

of insulin, which is required to clear all that sugar (glucose) from the blood. But this huge amount of insulin works too well, so within a couple of hours, your blood sugar level falls even lower than it was before you ate. Then your brain, the body's single biggest user of glucose, senses a decrease in fuel. So your brain responds by doing two things to restore normal blood sugar levels. It triggers the release of hormones to mobilize stored glucose and it sends out powerful signals to get more glucose into the system. Then the effect of low blood sugar is to cause you to eat again. It wouldn't be so bad if you ate the right foods, but you are looking for a quick fix to stop the hunger pangs so you grab a candy bar, a muffin, or even whole wheat crackers, and you start the process all over again.

If you start the day with eggs, lean ham and fresh strawberries, for example, and continue with ample amounts of protein and green vegetables at meals, you will burn fat all day long. The goal for maintaining a healthy weight and for weight-loss is to keep the body burning fat as much and as long as possible throughout the day. And don't worry; your body will do fine with this alternate energy source. Burning fat is normal and our bodies are very efficient at performing this function.

Here is a sample of an easy eating schedule that is simple to follow and portable so it convenient to carry with you throughout the day:

: **Protein drink and protein bar (like South Beach Brand), or cottage cheese and fruit, or**

yogurt with a ¼ oz of nuts and fruit.8 am

: Small can of tuna or string cheese and celery**10 am**

: **Large green salad with Chicken, or lean Ham. Dress with Seasoned Rice Vinegar. Low**

carb-high fiber wrap or tortilla1 pm,

: Protein shake or protein bar**3pm**

6pm: Lean ham slice rolled around string cheese.

8pm: 6 oz. Lean protein (chicken breast, pork loin, fish turkey, low-fat beef (sirloin) and large

serving of green vegetables (salad with tomatoes onion and bell pepper and green beans)

: **Low-fat (100 calories or less) Yogurt, pudding, or frozen fudge bar.10 pm**

As you can see, with this simple eating plan you eat all day long for under 1500 calories! Calories are important in that you need to have an idea of how many you are consuming in a day, but not so important that you have drive yourself crazy counting them.   Of course, you can add or

subtract food as you feel is best for you. The more you stay away from starches, sugars and refined carbohydrates, the more satisfied and successful you will be at maintaining or reducing your weight.

Keeping a supply of protein drinks and bars can be a huge benefit for ease and convenience. When you don't have time, or don't feel like having a meal, all you have to do is grab a drink or a bar and your body is getting the protein and nutrients it needs to function properly. You can always add more fresh vegetables to help keep you feeling satisfied. The crunchiness of cucumbers, carrots and celery seem to help satisfy the need to chew without adding unnecessary calories. You can also add fresh fruit like apples, bananas, strawberries, grapes, blueberries, etc. But the main idea that I want to get across to you is that you don't have to starve. You have a plethora of great options as food choices. As a mater of fact, it is very important to eat frequently throughout the day to keep your metabolism fired up and working.

Now for people who succeed with more structure and specific meal plans, I have included the following 2-Week Meal Plan to help guide you along and help you stay on track. Each day is roughly between 1200 and 1800 calories per day. These are simply guidelines, with no need to weigh or measure food. Some days you will eat more, other days you will eat less. None of us eat the same amount or eat in the same pattern every day. You know what an over-size portion of food looks like. If you want a larger portion, have it, but just make sure it's vegetables or fruit.

I drink coffee with real half& half and 'Equal'. A lot of plans steer clear of "real" cream, but I like it so I would rather give up "real" sugar. On this plan you can eat whatever you like, just reasonable amounts along with some kind of exercise most days of the week. I don't eat egg-substitutes or separated egg-whites, but if that is what you like, please feel free to enjoy those products.

I use real eggs, real butter and full-fat olive oil and salad dressings. I know what they are made of, they taste better and I can limit the amount I use so I still get the benefit of full flavor. The brands named are the ones I really use. All of the food on the following plan is as it is written, plain and simple. There are no recipes, only lists of ingredients. That way you can experiment with the ingredients, spices, and herbs. Besides if you cook like I do, you don't follow recipes too closely anyway. If there is no quantity listed next to the food item, you may have as much as you like. You can add all the spices and herbs that you like. Experiment with fresh herbs and various spices to add another dimension of flavor to any food. It's easy to get started and the food is good as well as healthy.

Day 1

Breakfast

2 Scrambled eggs with mushroom, red bell pepper, green onion and a sprinkle of grated cheese. 1 piece of whole wheat toast. Coffee or tea.

Lunch

Ham sandwich on Whole Grain Bread

Cucumber Slices

Diet Green Tea

Mid-afternoon snack

¼ cup dry roasted nuts

Dinner

6 oz. Salmon with baby greens. (I eat about 6 ounces of salmon. Most plans call for 4 ounces, but that is not enough protein for me to feel satisfied. Adjust the amount to suit you, but try not to exceed 6 ounces).

Bedtime Snack

1 carton of non-fat or low-fat, sugar-free yogurt.

Day 2

Breakfast

1 cup low-fat or non-fat cottage cheese

½ cup pineapple in natural juice

Coffee or tea

Lunch

1 Cup cooked Pinto beans

2 high fiber, low carb wraps

¼ cup Cheddar cheese

Salsa

Lettuce, Tomatoes, green Onions

Mid-afternoon Snack

1 carton low-fat, sugar-free yogurt

Dinner

6 Jumbo Shrimp sautéed in garlic, tomatoes, and fresh Basil and 1 Tbsp Olive Oil or Butter

1 Cup fresh green beans and red pepper slivers steamed in chicken broth and herbs

Tossed Salad with Rice Vinegar Vinaigrette

Bedtime Snack

2 containers fat-free, sugar-free pudding (100 calories or less)

Day 3

Breakfast

Rolls (4 oz turkey deli slices wrapped around 2, 80 calories string cheese sticks)

½ Cup strawberries

Coffee or tea

Mid-morning Snack

EAS 17-gram Protein Drink

Lunch

1 Lemon Chicken Breast cooked with garlic and capers

Tomato and cucumber slices with 2 Tbsps dressing of choice

Mid-afternoon Snack

Celery with 2Tbsps Peanut Butter

Dinner

1 Mediterranean Grilled Chicken Breast cooked in Olive oil with oregano, black olives, tomatoes, garlic

and capers

Grilled Asparagus

Tossed lettuce and Yellow tomato salad

Bedtime Snack

Skinny Cow Fudge Bar

Day 4

Breakfast

1 100-calorie English muffin, 1 Sausage Patty, 1 slice cheddar Cheese

Coffee or tea

Mid-morning Snack

1 pear

Baby Carrots

Lunch

Fajita Chicken Salad ; 1 sliced breast cooked with onion, red, orange, and green bell peppers served

on Large green Salad

1 low-carb, high fiber tortilla

Mid-afternoon Snack

" 100-calorie Protein bar

Dinner

1 small sirloin pork chop with Portobello mushrooms and onions

Baby Spinach sautéed in 1 TBl EVOO and 3 cloves fresh garlic

1 Large sliced tomato & fresh Basil drizzled with Balsamic Vinaigrette

Bedtime Snack

Fat-free Pudding

Day 5

Breakfast

6 Silver Dollar Pancakes (Aunt Jemima, frozen) with Light Butter syrup

2 slices Canadian bacon

Coffee or tea

Midmorning Snack

Cucumber and red bell pepper slices

Lunch

Tuna Salad on PumpernickelSandwich

Tomato and Lettuce

Baby carrots

Mid-afternoon Snack

Tangerine

Dinner

Lettuce Wrapped Turkey Tacos (6 oz ground , Romaine lettuce for wrappers)

Salsa, green onions, ¼ cup Cheddar Cheese, Chopped Tomatoes

Bedtime Snack

1 carton Fat-free, Sugar-free yogurt

Day 6

Breakfast

1 Chicken Breast on 2 slices 80-calorie Wheat bread

Coffee or tea

Mid-morning snack

Small Pear

Lunch

Tuna on Salad (1 6oz can water-packed tuna)

Large Lettuce and tomato salad with ½ apple and slivered almonds

Mid-afternoon Snack

Grape Tomatoes

Dinner

Herbed Chicken Breast

Garlic Green Beans

Large Tossed Salad with 2Tbsps Ranch Dressing

Bedtime Snack

1 carton Fat-free, Sugar-free Yogurt

Day 7

Breakfast

8 oz. low-fat Cottage Cheese

½ Cup Strawberries

Coffee or Tea

Midmorning Snack

Celery Sticks

Lunch

6-inch Subway Low-fat Chicken Sandwich

1 Bag of Apple Slices (sold at Subway)

Mid-afternoon snack

Sweet Mini-peppers

Dinner

Grilled Beef Kabobs (Beef cubes, onion, red & green bell peppers)

Large green salad with 2 Tbsps Dressing of Choice

Grilled Yellow Squash

Bedtime Snack

1 mini-bag Microwave Popcorn

Day 8

Breakfast

1 carton fat-free, sugar-free yogurt

1 140-calorie South Beach Protein Bar

Lunch

6 oz. Chicken Salad

2 Wasa Multi grain Crispbread Crackers

Grape Tomatoes

Mid-afternoon Snack

¼ Cup Dry-roasted Nuts

Dinner

6 oz Petit Sirloin Steak

Grilled Onions

Tossed Lettuce and Tomato Salad

Bedtime Snack

1 Pear

Day 9

Breakfast

½ Whole Grain Bagel

1 Tbsps Sugar-free Fruit Spread

Coffee or tea

Midmorning Snack

Cucumber Slices

Lunch

1/6 Digornio Vegetable Pizza

Small Tossed Salad

Mid-afternoon Snack

1 Cup Green or Red Grapes

Dinner

1 Chicken Breast on Large Green Salad

1 Cup steamed Yellow squash

Bedtime Snack

Celery Sticks

Day 10

Breakfast

1 100-calorie English muffin

1 tsp. Peanut Butter and 1 tsp fruit Spread

Coffee or tea

Midmorning Snack

1 medium Apple

Lunch

1 and Cheese 'Lean Pocket'

Lettuce and Tomato Salad

Mid-afternoon Snack

10 Large Black or Green Olives

Dinner

6 oz Sirloin Pork Chop Stir-fry with onions, red bell pepper, green onions, and bamboo shoots

Steamed broccoli

Bedtime Snack

1 carton fat-free, sugar-free pudding

Day 11

Breakfast

2 Scrambled eggs with 1 slice deli ham

1 Tangerine

Coffee or tea

Midmorning Snack

1 carton Fat-free, Sugar-free Yogurt

Lunch

Turkey Burger, No bun, with lettuce, tomato, onion, mustard, relish, and ketchup

Celery stalks, Green Pepper Rings with 1 Tbsps Ranch Dressing for dipping

Mid-afternoon Snack

¼ Cup dry-roasted nuts

Dinner

Shrimp and Broccoli Stir-fry (6 Jumbo Shrimp with 5-spice seasoning)

Large Spinach Salad (2 Cups) with Fat-free Oriental Dressing

Bedtime Snack

4 oz Fat-free Cottage Cheese

Day 12

Breakfast

2 oz Deli ham, 1 hard-boiled egg, 1 low-fat string cheese stick

Coffee or tea

Mid-morning Snack

Cucumber Slices

Lunch

1 Cup Cuban Black Bean Soup

1 High Fiber, Low Carb tortilla

¼ Cup Cheddar Cheese

Mid-afternoon Snack

Baby Carrots

Dinner

1 Broiled Chicken Breast

Lemon Pepper Green Beans

Lettuce and Tomato Salad

Bedtime Snack

1 Medium Peach

Day 13

Breakfast

1 EAS Protein Drink (110 calories)

1 South Beach Meal Replacement Bar (180 calories, 12 grams Protein)

Coffee or tea

Midmorning Snack

Grape Tomatoes

Lunch

1 Chicken Breast on top of   Large Spinach Salad

5 Black Olives, Diced Tomato, and 1 tsp Feta Cheese

Balsamic Dressing

Mid-afternoon Snack

Red and Green Bell pepper rings

Dinner

6 oz Salmon baked in salsa with cilantro and green onions

Sliced tomato and Lettuce salad with Lime Vinaigrette

Bedtime Snack

Skinny Cow Ice cream Sandwich

Day 14

Breakfast

1 Cup low-fat Cottage Cheese

4 oz pineapple tidbits in natural juice

1 slice 80-calorie wheat toast

Coffee or tea

Midmorning Snack

¼ Cup Pecans

Lunch

Taco Salad (6oz ground meat on top of Mixed Greens)

Salsa, Onions, chopped black olives, ¼ cup cheddar cheese

10 Tortilla Chips

Mid-afternoon Snack

Strawberries

Dinner

Chicken Scampi (1 chicken breast cooked with garlic and 2 Tbsps Butter, and 1 oz white wine)

Wilted Spinach

Sliced Tomato and Fresh Basil Salad

Bedtime Snack

1 carton fat-free, sugar-free pudding

So there you have it, a simple, 2-week eating plan that is packed with lots of food choices and lots of flavor. Once you start eating healthier foods, you'll find that it's really not that hard and you will automatically start to pay more attention to what you put into your mouth. The goal is not perfection, because we all "fall off the wagon" at one time or another. The goal is to eat healthier *most of the time. Once you reach your health goals, I'm sure you'll find changing your eating habits was definitely worth the effort. Good Luck!*

Chapter 7: Why Vitamins are Vital

Read enough nutrition news and you will see that not all scientists agree on multivitamins. There ha

ve always been two schools of thought regarding the need for vitamins as an adjunct to fitness and

good health.   One school supports the use of vitamins as a supplement to an adequate food intake,

and the other school believes vitamin supplements are completely unnecessary. Looking at all the

evidence it appears that taking a daily vitamin is safe and beneficial for most people. Whichever way

you think, there is plenty of research based information available to help you make the decision that is best for you. Personally, I am an advocate of vitamins and take one most days.

They are not magic pill, but a lack of vitamins can cause fatigue, especially B vitamins, which convert energy from food into energy your body can use. If you are not getting enough nutrient power in your diet, a multivitamin could help.

For decades researchers were divided on the value of taking a multivitamin. Now there is a growing consensus that taking a daily vitamin is a great nutrition insurance policy that may auqment your daily diet.   In an article from the Harvard School of public Health written in 2013, the message was simple: a daily vitamin and an extra Vitamin D supplement is a good way to make sure you are getting all the nutrients you need to be healthy.

Vitamins are difficult to classify. They are not fat, carbohydrate or protein and they do n ot supply calories. Vitamins do not produce energy; instead they are catalysts that spark the assimilation of other nutrients. They are organic molecules necessary for facilitating the chemical reactions and for building molecules in the body that are vital to health. Vitamins are essential in varying quantities as links in the metabolism of other nutrients to maintain bodily functions. No one food contains all the vitamins necessary for optimal growth and body maintenance

Incredible as it may seem today, vitamins were only discovered in the early 1900's. Their discovery had significant implications on mankind's understanding of health and wellness. Researcher s learned that vitamins were not only necessary for life, but that not having enough of them contributed to major diseases. By 1930, the U.S. government had published its first "Recommended Daily Allowances" to establish potency levels for 12 vitamins and eight essential minerals. As a result il lnesses such as scurvy, pellagra, and rickets were virtually eliminated.
Within 10 years, doctors were seeing such overall health improvements in people of all ages that they began to examine the positive effects of vitamin and mineral supplements. They discovered the power of vitamins could not only prevent malnutrition but could also heal physical ailments as well.

In the past experts claimed if people ate healthy diets, taking vitamins was unnecessary. However research now demonstrates it is beneficial for the majority of adults to take a multivitamin every day. Scientists have discovered evidence showing vitamins not only keep away deficiency diseases but may also avert the onset of chronic diseases including cancer, heart disease, and osteoporosis.

An unhealthy diet cannot be remedied by taking a daily vitamin. Multivitamins only provide a minute quantity of nutrients that work in conjunction with the food we eat. Generally speaking, vitamin supplements should be regarded as nutritional "backup". There have been previous studies suggesting that a multivitamin daily is especially beneficial to the elderly in helping that population more disease resistant.

Although everyone over 18 is considered an adult, the nutritional needs of a 20 year old are quite different than the needs of a75 year old. People of different ages and different stages of life have different vitamin needs as well. For example, after age 50 the body needs more vitamin D to efficiently absorb calcium which helps prevent osteo porosis. Most people are not aware of the body's changing nutrient requirements throughout adulthood. Vitamins are essential to all bodily processes. Each one of us has a unique physical composition and unique nutritional needs.

The final decision regarding the use of vitamin supplements is a personal choice that should be made with regards to the most up to date research information available.

There are 5 vitamins that play a key role in maintaining optimal health which in turn, contributes to overall fitness. These five vitamins are:
1. Folic Acid
2. Vitamin B 12
3. Vitamin B 6
4. Vitamin D
5. Vitamin C

The B vitamins are important multi-taskers. They aid in the metabolism of carbohydrates, fats and proteins, assist in the growth and repair of tissues, and enhance our sense of well-being and clear thinking by supporting our nervous system.

Biotin, one of the B vitamins, has been found to help with drowsiness. The most efficient way to take these vitamins is as a compound such as B-complex.

Recent research is also linking two additional B vitamins and folic acid in the fight against various types of cancer and heart disease. After 2 children died of massive strokes in 1968, a Boston pathologist began to study a protein breakdown by-product known as homocysteine found in their bodies. Following the initial study, subsequent research has connected high levels of homocysteine to increased risk for stroke and heart disease. Vitamins B6, B12, and Folic Acid have been found to help recycle homocysteine into one of 20 chemicals the body uses to create new proteins. If the body is deficient in B vitamins or Folic Acid, the homocysteine cannot be converted and levels increase causing an increased risk for stroke and heart disease. In addition, Folic acid has been found to lessen depression by indirectly aiding in the production of neurotransmitters such as serotonin and dopamine which help regulate mood, sleep, and appetite. Folic acid in combination with certain B vitamins has also been linked to the fight against various types of cancer and heart disease.

Although the exact optimal daily intake of these vitamins is unknown, researchers believe very few adults get the adequate amount. In the past deficiencies of these vitamins was the cause of pernicious anemia, a fatal disease that plagued its victims with disorientation, hallucinations, tingling in the extremities and memory loss. Today the disease is no longer common and those affected are ea sily and successfully treated with a combination of B vitamins.

Vitamin D is the new super-nutrient. In the past few years there has been an explosion of research on its far-reaching benefits for all age groups. The most remarkable benefits of vitamin D are; It helps decrease blood sugar, it helps maintain healthy blood pressure, it helps decrease inflammation, it helps prevent the abnormal growth of unwanted blood vessels found in cancer and macular degeneration, it helps preserve muscle strength and function, it helps fortify calcium intake and it's great for bone health. It helps maintain grip strength, protects against fibromyalgia, multiple sclerosis, and depression. Vitamin D is also an immune system booster, helps with cell growth, and helps prevent melanoma or non-Hodgskin's lymphoma.

Vitamin D promotes healthy bones and teeth and helps the body absorb calcium and phosphorus. Recent research has linked the lack of Vitamin D to certain forms of cancer. Vitamin D is converted by the liver into its active form, a hormone known as calcitrol that regulate calcium balance in the body. Research in Japan has found that the hormone suppresses leukemia cells by causing them to be turned into noncancerous cells. Additional studies conducted in laboratory setting found that Vitamin D blocked the cell division and growth in certain other types of cancer cells.

Until recent years, vitamin D deficiency was thought to be as rare as the bubonic plague, eradicated long ago by D- fortified foods such as milk. But in the past few years researchers and clinicians have become concerned that vitamin D deficiency may be a hidden problem among the nation's elderly population.

One researcher called it an "unrecognized epidemic" and it may be implicated in hip fractures

associated with advanced age   Vitamin D is not naturally found in many foods. It is produced in the

body by exposure to direct sunlight. Aim for consuming two foods daily containing vitamin D2 or D3. V

itamin D deficiency is most common in the northern most regions of the U.S. and in those individuals

who spend less than fifteen minutes a day in sunlight. An association between an increased risk of

bone fractures and Vitamin D deficiency has been established in multiple studies. Daily Vitamin D

supplement in those over the age of 50 is thought to decrease the risk of fractures. Take a vitamin D3

supplement daily, with teens and older adults aiming for 600 to 2000 IU of supplemental D3 daily.

The nutritional element known as vitamin C is one of the most important things to include in a

regular diet. This powerful vitamin provides a number of very important health benefits, and the body

needs it to function well. Vitamin C aids in staving off all kinds of diseases, improving the immune

system, preventing inflammation, and generally supplying the body with chemicals that help it to

process a diverse diet.

We've all heard about the old stories of how mariners used vitamin C to prevent the nefarious ailment called "scurvy" – but that age-old tale, for many, helps to illustrate how vitamin C can be an essential part of any diet. Without vitamin C, the bodies of these deprived sailors suffered. The same is true for a modern vitamin C deficiency. Individuals with this kind of vitamin deficiency become tired and experience various problems like gum disease, hair loss, etc.

So what is so important about this essential vitamin? Vitamin C contains antioxidants, which help fight off free radicals in the body, warding off inflammation, infections, and viruses. Furthermore, by helping to build proteins in various types of cellular constructions, vitamin C also protects against heart attacks and strokes. In general, this nutritional element promotes better vascular health and longevity. New studies have shown even more significant health benefits of vitamin C, where the vitamin has proved to be useful in breaking down some kinds of oxidized fats. This suggests that vitamin C may even be important in preventing things like Alzheimer's disease or autoimmune problems, as well as atherosclerosis, another problem of the circulatory system.

Doctors are often well versed about how this simple vitamin can affect multiple body processes. One specific manifestation of vitamin C effects is in its promotion of healthy teeth and gums. Periodontal problems and other related issues can be curbed with large intakes of vitamin C, although many other factors also apply. Generally, getting your daily recommended dose of vitamin C helps the body to handle challenges and build healthy tissues, while using the natural antioxidants to protect the body from outside invaders.

A variety of fresh fruits and vegetables contain a large amount of vitamin C. Citrus fruits are famous for including vitamin C, and shoppers buy oranges, lemons and limes by the bag in order to get vitamin C into their diet. However, cooking or processing will deplete some of the vitamin C that needs to be ingested by the body – that's why many individuals choose to take vitamin C tablets or supplements to be sure that they are getting their share of this wonderful health booster. For more information on how vitamin C intake could relate to any of your particular health issues, talk to your doctor about how a natural vitamin regimen can increase your overall health and quality of life.

Vitamin C is also known as ascorbic acid and was once thought to be a "cure-all" from the common cold to cancer. Vitamin C is required by the body for synthesis of neurotransmitters, hormones, carnitine, and collagen in connective tissue and for the conversion of cholesterol into bile salts. It also enhances the bioavailability of iron which helps absorption. Vitamin C is also a powerful antioxidant that protects the body against pollutants and free radicals. It is also linked to the prevention of degenerative diseases such as cataracts, certain cancers and cardiovascular diseases.

Ascorbic acid also promotes healthy cell development, proper calcium absorption, normal tissue growth and repair, especially in the healing of wounds and burns. It also assists in the prevention of blood clots and bruise and accumulates in white blood cells to maintain a strong immune response. Vitamin C is needed for healthy gums, to protect the body from infection. With all those important functions, no wonder Vitamin C has earned respect in the medical and nutritional communities.

The need for vitamin C is dramatically increased any time the body is subjected to stress such as st renuous exercise, trauma, infections, and elevated environmental temperatures. Since Vitamin C is a water soluble vitamin, it is not stored in the body and any excess is excreted in the urine. Good food sources of vitamin are green leafy vegetables, citrus fruits, tomatoes, melons, papayas, and strawberries.

Chapter 8: Rejuvenate with Rest

It may sound like a paradox, but rest is just as important as movement in order to maintain an active , healthy lifestyle. Rest repairs and renews the body and mind. Rest and sleep give our entire being a "mini-vacation". Sleep is something we do all throughcut our lives, a natural body function that most of us don't really think about. The truth is, sleep is vital to physical health and emotional well-being.

A good night's rest improves concentration and memory function, allows the body to repair any cell damage that occurred during the day, and strengthens the immune system which helps prevent disease. Sleep is a necessary time of renewal and directly relates to the way we feel

Sleep is still a mystery. Researchers have not been able to pinpoint the reasons that we sleep. Sleep is the ultimate research topic. Although much more is known about sleep today than 20 years ago, research on the subject of sleep is still growing. The amount of sleep you get and the quality of that sleep is more important than previously thought. It is well known that lack of sleep is attributed to less than "clear" thinking and poor concentration. It is now known that chronic lack of sleep can be a contributing factor in obesity and Type II diabetes.

According to research studies on sleep, it seems that "Sleeping Beauty" was on to something. As it turns out, sleep is just as essential as food, air, and water. Sleep is a restorative process. During sleep, growth hormone is released which is crucial to the maintenance of physical and mental balance. Sleep enhances the brain's ability to remember by enabling the brain to encode and store recently received information. REM sleep activates the areas of the brain responsible for learning. While we sleep, various parts of the brain responsible for emotions, decision-making, and social interaction are allowed to slow down. Rest for these areas of the brain during sleep allows optimal performance while awake. Neurons in the brain regenerate and repair during sleep, allowing our bodies to function more efficiently during waking hours. Research suggests that "deep sleep" allows for more antibody production and stimulates the immune system. Antibodies keep level of bacteria in our systems in check and help keep the body free of disease. Without proper sleep, the immune system can become weakened which leaves the body vulnerable to infection and disease. During sleep, cell production increases while proteins break down at a slower rate.

While lack of sleep can have dire consequences, adequate sleep provides only positive, healthful benefits. In a typical day, a person's waking hours are consumed trying to meet the many mental and physical demands encountered at every turn, as well as replenishing vital nutrients as they are being used up during these daily activities. In the hours remaining during sleep, the body takes time out to rebuild and recharge, preparing for the day ahead.

Electrical activity measured in the brain during sleep indicates that healthful physiological changes occur in 90-minute periods throughout the night, which means that the active biological clock in a person is set to operate in a circadian rhythm of 90-minute cycles that repeats every 25 to 28 hours. This clock is set and reset according to the amount of natural daylight available each day, thus evening sleep begins later in summer than in winter.

Losing sleep during any 24- or 48-hour period interferes with the essential and healthful cycle of physiological changes that occur during sleep and is detrimental to both physical and mental recovery. Recovery in subjects deprived of sleep for 24 hours has been measured at 72%, while recovery after a 48-hour period without sleep further deteriorated to a level of only 42%.2

Other clock-like rhythms occur between 3:00 a.m. and 6:00 a.m. and from 3:00 a.m. to 6:00 p.m., when our body temperature dips a degree or two and drowsiness results. We have all experienced this mid- or late-afternoon slump. In contrast, when body temperature peaks between 6:00 and 9:00p.m., we may become aware of a heightened sense of alertness. Then, as we tend to wind down from our daily activities sometime after 9:00 p.m., our body temperature falls again, and we are lulled into a state of drowsiness during which the brain converts low-voltage "beta" waves into higher voltage "alpha" waves.

As these alpha waves are, in turn, converted to slower " theta" waves during what are known as sleep stages 1 and 2, the skeletal muscles relax, causing the " hypnotic jerk" or "nodding" experience. When nodding off is not resisted or interrupted, the theta waves soon turn into even slower "delta" waves of the third and fourth stages of deeper sleep. During these stages, rapid-eye-movement {REM} sleep, dreams, and actual muscle paralysis take place. If, for some reason, muscle paralysis does not occur, the vividness of the dream state will physically draw the dreamer into an active state of sleepwalking or, worse yet, intense physical activity that will further break down exhausted muscle tissues already in need of repair.

During undisturbed sleep or slow-wave sleep, the plasma growth hormone (human growth hormone - somatropin -) in humans is found to be at its highest levels. If the sleep stage process is interrupted, complete repair of soft tissues is impossible due to the resulting decrease or absence of human growth hormone - somatropin - .

Noise pollution has been shown to have a dramatic effect on a person's optimal sleep. Aircraft noise endured by those living in homes near airports can reach a level of 55 to 75 decibels inside the homes. Significant noise such as this has been observed to raise the adrenaline and noradrenaline levels of all those sampled during sleep, an effect which is detrimental to achieving normal, healthy, recuperative sleep. Exposure to high levels of noise during the day can also interfere with getting a sound night's sleep. Daytime noise pollution of 80 decibels or more tends to elevate both heart and respiration rates, which may further disrupt full-stage, recuperative sleep.

Another component of ensuring a good night's sleep is to maintain a balanced ratio of macro- and micronutrients. What we eat and drink has a remarkable influence upon our sleep. Relatively small amounts of alcohol, as little as 0.8 grams per kilogram body weight, will suppress plasma growth hormone values as much as 75% when consumed just prior to sleep.

The bottom line is that when sleep is altered (reduced or extended), performance and mood are both affected. Altered sleep time by delaying, extending, or advancing each phase of slumber by a 3-hour time span. Achieving that elusive perfect night's sleep, then, would seem to depend upon enjoying a low-key day in a stress-free environment followed by seeking sleep at a routine time in a quiet, totally dark room.

Generally speaking, we tend to feel more receptive to sleep when it is dark outside or when we are in a darkened room, and we feel an awakening when we are immersed in light. The famous artist Claude Monet once described nightfall as a time of "mini-death". The brain's pineal gland regulates the hormonal effects of light's influence on body cycles, mood eating and sleeping patterns, and activity levels. This gland is responsible for the secretion of the hormone melatonin, which is released at night and inhibited during the day.

The appearance of skin, eyes, and facial complexion reflect the body's inner state of being. Sleep can be regarded as cosmetic medicine because it acts as a natural "anti-aging" solution.

The body enters a maintenance and repair state while we sleep. This is the primary reason many dermatologists recommend using an active skin cream at bedtime.

At its most fundamental level sleep seems to be a metabolic imperative. When we are awake the body's cells are breaking down to support mobility, nutrition, and basic daily function. The wakeful state is stressful and after a certain number of hours, the body must return to sleep. It is during sleep damage is repaired, growth takes place, and the immune system actively protects the body from viruses and foreign organisms that may have invaded the body during the day.

During the day our bodies are exposed to a host of elements such as stress, pollution, and UV rays that contribute to the aging process. Sleep is the time-out the body needs to make necessary cellular repairs and restore itself from the inside out. Deep sleep acts as our private operating room for all the "nips and tucks" that occur within our bodies during this type of sleep. This is the time the body uses for skin repair, new cell growth, and fortification against moisture loss and free radical damage. Many cells also increase production of proteins which become building blocks needed for cell growth and cell damage repair. For this reason deep sleep is synonymous with "beauty sleep".

As your skin dries out throughout the day, moisture is lost and stretched out skin falls into wrinkles. As you sleep, the body lowers its temperature by perspiring. This perspiration helps replace moisture in the top layers of skin and fills skin cells. Creams or lotions applied to the skin before sleep h elps to fill the top layer of skin cells and makes the skin look smoother and fuller.

Topical products may not be incorporated at the cellular level. These products may improve the appearance of the skin by "plumping up' the cells. A better method to accomplish the same goal is to nourish and hydrate our skin from the inside out. Through sleep, our bodies are able to use its own nutrients and collagen building capacities. Sleep is own personal airbrush. Overnight skin repair is the body's all-natural weapon against aging and the onset of wrinkles.

Six Reasons to Get Enough Sleep

1. **Learning and memory**: Sleep helps the brain commit new information to memory through

a process called memory consolidation. In studies, people who'd slept after learning a task did

better on tests later.

2. **Metabolism and weight**: Chronic sleep deprivation may cause weight gain by affecting the

way our bodies process and store carbohydrates, and by altering levels of hormones that

affect our appetite.

3. **Safety**: Sleep debt contributes to a greater tendency to fall asleep during the daytime.

These lapses may cause falls and mistakes such as medical errors, air traffic mishaps, and

road accidents.

4. Mood: Sleep loss may result in irritability, impatience, inability to concentrate, and moodiness. Too little sleep can also leave you too tired to do the things you like to do.

5. Cardiovascular health: Serious sleep disorders have been linked to hypertension, increased stress hormone levels, and irregular heartbeat.

6. Disease: Sleep deprivation alters immune function, including the activity of the body's killer cells. Keeping up with sleep may also help fight cancer.

Sleep is a necessity, not a luxury. Once regarded as non-productive function of unconscious activity, sleep is now regarded as a "rejuvenation" period for the mind and body. It took a while before researchers invested in the study of sleep. However, in the last 40 years, sleep research has gone full bore with new research being conducted continually and sleep-study clinics gaining popularity nationwide.

Neurologists have proven that sleep is not a passive state, but rather an elaborate activity with its own specific functions necessary for physical and mental health. Sleep loss can have profound detrimental effects on mood, thinking, productivity, communication, and physical performance. The rhythmic patterns of sleep and dreaming that repeat themselves throughout the night serve as the brain's "filling station". As we sleep, there are dramatic changes in body temperature, respirations, and heart rate. With an adequate amount of sleep, we have an opportunity to perform at our peak level each day.

Chapter 9: Maintain Your Brain

We can choose to maintain mental fitness and agility as a way of slowing down the aging process. Current research shows that most negative changes associated with aging can be successfully prevented and sometimes treated. Researchers are beginning to agree that taking care of your general health may help your long term brain function. Total brain health begins with proper nutrition, brain-stimulating activity and physical exercise.

Mental fitness is closely tied to the health of all organs and systems. If the brain does not function at a sufficient level, life cannot continue. Over 100 billion neurons form over a trillion connections in the brain which are fed by blood circulating throughout the body. The heart, blood vessels and immune system, all have tremendous influence on brain function. The brain consumes about 20 percent of the oxygen taken into the body and about 25 percent of the body's glucose to sustain baseline function.

The brain is a remarkable organ that can be repaired and strengthened throughout our lifetime. The brain is responsible for all intelligent thought. It reasons, makes rational decisions, learns information, stores information, and retrieves information as needed. The right and left sides of the brain are equal in size, but in most people, one side is dominant which produces distinct personality traits. Left-brained people tend to be talented in science, math, reading, and verbal communication. Their decisions are guided by logic or reasoning. Right –brained individuals are often insightful, creative, perceptive, artistic, and socially oriented. Their decisions are often guided by emotion and intuition. A person is said to have a well integrated brain when the intellectual and the emotional functions are balanced and well incorporated.

By age 50, most people experience a 10 to 20 percent drop in blood flow to the brain. This drop continues as people age, which results in fewer nutrients being delivered to the brain cells. Insufficient blood flow can be the outcome of poor circulatory health due to physical inactivity, obesity, diabetes, and cardiovascular disease. Although scientists acknowledge that genes play an important role in predetermining your brain's aging, researchers agree that taking care of your health may enhance long term brain function.

Breakthrough   research indicates that our brains continue to make new connections well into advanced age, emphasizing the importance of nurturing mental activity throughout our lives. The mental decline associated with aging appears largely due to altered connections among brain cells. Studies conclude that keeping the brain active seems to increase its ability to build and generate new cells.

Scientists are making significant progress in understanding what constitutes normal brain aging. Contrary to earlier beliefs, decline in neuron number is not significantly involved in normal brain aging. In fact, recent evidence indicates the older brain is capable of generating new nerve cells in the hippocampus area of the brain which is largely responsible for acquiring and processing information. B y remaining connected and engaged in social, family, and community activities one can achieve and maintain optimal brain function. The aging brain maintains the capacity to make new connections, absorb new information, and acquire new skills.

The more we use our mental capacities, the stronger they will be. Mentally stimulating activity strengthens brain cells and the connections between them. There are many brain stimulating activities we can incorporate into our daily lives. As we get older, we need to deliberately challenge our brains. Scientists suggest trying to memorize names, addresses, and telephone numbers as a way of improving the working memory. Trivia games, brain teasers, crossword puzzles, and trying new hobbies are excellent ways to get mental exercise and flex your brain's muscle.

Successful aging studies have consistently shown that a higher level of physical activity correlates with better brain function. Current research shows that most of the negative changes that occur with aging can be successfully prevented and treated, in some cases. And though scientists acknowledge that genes play a large role in predetermining brain aging, researchers agree that maintaining general health might also enhance long-term brain function. Total brain health begins with proper nutrition, brain- stimulating activity, and physical activity. Physical exercise plays an important role in mental acuity.

Mental fitness is closely tied to the health of the other organs and systems in the body. The heart, immune, and circulatory systems have tremendous influence on brain function. Slow, progressive decline in cognitive functions is a natural process of aging. Recently thousands of published studies have determined that a certain amount of cognitive decline can be controlled. Some studies demonstrate preventative measures will help maintain optimal brain function. Recently, thousands of published studies indicate our brains continue to make new connections well into advanced age.

The mental decline associated with aging appears to be due, in large part, to altered connections among brain cells. Studies conclude keeping the brain active increases its vitality and may help build and generate new brain cells. Without the debilitating effects of disease, older people can maintain mental acuity by participating in activities that stimulate the mind and body. Severe mental decline is not inevitable; the aging brain maintains the capacity to absorb new information, acquire new skills, and make new connections.

Contrary to earlier beliefs, decline in neuron number is not significantly involved in normal brain aging. Recent evidence indicates the older brain is capable of generating new nerve cells, particularly in the area of the brain important for acquiring and processing information, the hippocampus. Therefore, if the brain remains healthy and disease free it should continue to function normally, maintain connections, and build new networks throughout our lives.

Maintaining a healthy cardiovascular system ensures proper blood flow to the brain supplying it with the fundamental component needed to function optimally. Physical activity oxygenates the blood, supports good blood flow to the brain and encourages the formation of new brain cells. Exercise increases levels of brain chemicals that encourage the formation of new brain cells. Physical activity also helps maintain brain structure and function and may delay the onset of Alzheimer's disease and other dementias.

There is a large body of evidence that suggests exercise has enhanced beneficial effects on the brain from middle to old age. Clinical data revealed that people who exercise several times a week show decreased cognitive decline compared with those who have a low level of physical activity. Clinical studies also link fitness training to improved cognition, increased brain efficiency, and prevention of brain atrophy in the elderly. By strengthening the link between your body and brain, you will improve the chances of maintaining your mental edge.

The brain responds to new and novel experiences by releasing a rush of neurotransmitters, such as dopamine, which makes you more alert. There is no need to do anything drastic. Just take an ordinary task or routine, and switch it up. As an example, if you are right handed, use the left hand to brush your teeth.

The midlife years offer fresh learning opportunities. Rich undeveloped and underdeveloped capacities are often tapped during this stage of life. Albert Einstein took up playing the violin late in life and Winston Churchill took up painting. Any stage of life is a good time to launch a new interest. You will gain increased knowledge, a renewed sense of accomplishment, and better brain function as a result of trying "something new". Here is a list of brain-stimulating activities to consider:

1) Start a journal of appreciation. Every day write down all the things in your life that you are thankful for. When you see the words, you will realize how fortunate you are.

2) Take a Picture. Photography can be a creative outlet that gets you out and about and helps change the observers focus.

3) Go Window Shopping. Go into a store you have never been in and absorb the sights, sounds, and smells of the experience. Get some great ideas for fashion or decorating to incorporate into your style.

4) Try a new recipe. Give your taste buds a treat. Making up recipes is a wonderful way to express creativity and have fun.

5) Read a Good Book. Let your imagination run wild and "vacation" from your current reality temporarily. Reading is a great brain-stimulating activity in many ways.

Using the brain's cognitive capacities strengthens and maintains them. Mentally stimulating activity strengthens the brain cells and the connections between them. The more the mental capacities are used, the stronger they become. Research recommends exercising the brain 50 hours a month, which translates to about 2 hours a day. Regular challenges to the brain help retain cognitive abilities and mental acuity.

There are many activities that we can incorporate into our daily lives to help maintain better brain health and ensure peak mental performance. To improve working memory, scientists suggest trying to memorize names, addresses, and phone numbers instead of relying on devices in which the information is stored. Trivia games, brain teasers' reading, writing, crossword puzzles, and trying new hobbies are excellent ways to get mental exercise and flex your brain's muscle. According to research, when you continue to exercise your brain from an early age, your intellectual powers can be at a peak during the middle years. With continued challenges there is great potential for the energies and creativity of the brain to continue at high levels long after the body has slowed down.

Successful aging studies have consistently shown that higher levels of physical activity are associated with better brain aging. Physical activity helps maintain a healthy cardiovascular system which ensures proper blood flow to the brain supplying it with the raw material it needs to perform properly. Physical activity oxygenates the blood and maintains good circulation to the brain, which encourages the formation of new brain cells. Exercise increases the levels of brain chemicals that promote the growth of nerve cells. Physical activity also helps maintain brain structure and my delay the onset of some dementias.

Clinical data demonstrates that people who exercise several times a week show a reduced rate of cognitive decline compared with those who have low levels of physical activity. Clinical trials also suggest a relationship between physical activity and increased brain efficiency, as well as prevention of brain atrophy in the elderly. In a 4 year study of subjects from 62 to 70years old revealed that the subjects who were employed and exercised regularly had sustained levels of cerebral blood flow and superior performance on cognitive tests compared to inactive people in the same age group.

Current data indicates all level of physical activity benefit brain activity, although an exact amount is unknown. Based on clinical findings of exercising older (60+) adults, exercising 3 or more times a week for 30 to 45 minutes seemed to benefit brain function. Unstructured physical activity such as walking around the block, walking a mall or major "big box" store can be easily included into a daily routine.

Eating a brain-healthy diet can help reduce the risk of Alzheimer's dementia, cardiovascular disease, and diabetes by maintaining adequate blood flow to the brain. Fresh vegetables, fruits, and fish high in omega 3 and omega6 are considered heart and brain healthy foods. By recognizing the link between your diet and your brain, you can maintain and enhance your mental edge. The biochemicals responsible for brain function come indirectly from the foods we eat. When we eat for optimal health, we maximize our chances for the most advantageous brain function.

Of the 4 essential nutrient groups, the most important to brain chemistry are amino acids, which are the building blocks of protein. Amino acids serve familiar nutritional roles that sustain every aspect of health. Amino acids are the precursors to neurotransmitters which are chemical messengers that help relay information throughout the body. There are approximately 22 amino acids together in various combinations that create all the structural proteins of the body. The body manufactures 14 of the 22, but the remaining eight are considered essential because the body cannot manufacture them and must come from the food we eat. Amino acids are found in foods such as meats, poultry, eggs, fish, cheese, and seeds. The eight essential amino acids are: Isoleucine, Leucine, Lysine, Methionine, Phenylalanine, Threonine, Typtophan and Valine.

Isoleucine and Leucine are two of the amino acids that make up 1/3 of your muscle tissue. They provide muscle fuel, making them a common supplement for athletes. In addition, Isoleucine is a necessary part of hemoglobin, the oxygen carrying protein in red blood cells. Both amino acids help muscles recover from strenuous activity and boost endurance.

Lysine is needed for the intestinal absorption of calcium and is necessary for collagen formation, a protein that makes up your bones, ligaments, cartilage, and tendons. In conjunction with vitamin C, lysine produces hydroxylysine, a substance incorporated into collagen. It also helps produce antibodies, making it an important part of the immune system. Methionine is also involved in collagen production and has the added function of helping the liver metabolize fats. Methionine is an antioxidant the body uses to neutralize and prevent damage by free radicals.

Phenylalanine plays a crucial role in producing important brain chemicals. The body converts phenylalanine to another amino acid called tyrosine. Tyrosine is responsible for manufacturing epinephrine, norepinephrine and thyroid hormones, which are the chemicals that regulate mood, appetite, metabolism, and sleep-wake cycles. Threorine helps the body stabilize blood sugar and is necessary for the formation of tooth enamel, collagen, and elastin, a substance that contributes to muscle, skin, and tendon flexibility.

The last of the eight essential amino acids are tryptophan and Valine. Tryptophan's primary function is to produce serotonin, brain chemical involved in mood regulation. A deficiency of serotonin contributes to depression and anxiety. Valine is responsible for promoting growth, tissue repair, and blood sugar regulation.

The ancient Romans were extremely accurate in the famous quote, "Mens sana in copore sano", which translates to "healthy mind in a healthy body". The first steps to maintaining a healthy brain and body to concentrate on a diet rich in fruits, vegetables, plant-proteins, whole-grains, and oily cold-water fish. These foods contain large amounts of brain-boosting ingredients such as antioxidants, omega-3 fatty acids and other significant natural compounds. In a study conducted by the Agriculture Research Service antioxidants were shown to counter brain decline and actually "turn back the clock" to some extent. Your brain cells need a high intake of antioxidants like the vitamin E family compounds found in the germ of whole grains, the vitamin C found in citrus fruits, and the Carotenoids found in red and orange vegetables.

Chapter 10: Satisfy Your Soul

Our soul is the deepest essence of whom and what we are. Our soul is where the *real you resides. Your soul knows your deepest joys and carries your wounds. Your soul harbors the potential for growth, change, and honesty. The soul's purpose in our lives is to allow us to experience spiritual growth. Through our soul work, we learn to transcend the world as we know it. Through exploring the depths of our souls we come to better understand the true meaning of our lives.*

As a result of life experience, two major developments occur as we age. We become more aware of changes deep inside that lead us to spiritual growth. During our youth we rarely consider our inner life, as we are primarily interested and immersed in the world around us. As we age and gain life experience, our priorities change and we perceive our lives differently. Background aspects of life come into sharper focus, while others we once focused on so strongly, fade away. We begin to feel connected to others and we begin to experience life in a way we never have before.

We need to make time thinking about our souls and finding ways to nurture the wonderful feelings that come forth when we feed our souls. "Soul food" is whatever makes you feel alive, whole, and satisfied deep inside. Soul food is whatever brings a sense of inner peace and a feeling of well-being. Everyone's soul food is different. Some common sources of soul are; art, nature, music, and dancing. Some uncommon, sources of soul food are gratitude, compassion, humility, and generosity.

Nurturing the soul needs to be a lifelong process that frames life changes as continued opportunities for spiritual growth. Despite inevitable losses, life does bear unexpected fruits. This is a process of acknowledgment, reconciliation, and peace. Nurturing the soul is a time to express gratitude for all the blessings we have received while living our lives with intention, joy, and appreciation.

Being a "spiritual" being has many meanings. It is not necessarily reflected in any commitment to an organized religion, and we know that many outwardly pious people are the least spiritual. Spirituality means the acceptance of what is. Spirituality means the ability to find peace and happiness in an imperfect world, and to feel that one's own personality is imperfect but acceptable. Fro m this peaceful state of mind comes the ability to love unconditionally. Acceptance, faith, love, and peace are some of the traits the define spirituality.

Spirituality is personal in its meaning to each individual. Doctrine has no meaning in a spiritual sense. Spirituality is a personal discovery, made alone over time. When you find out what it means to you, it will speak to you. For some, spirituality is achieved through religion and prayer. For others it involves being immersed in meditation, music, or yoga. And for others spirituality is experienced when communing with nature; a walk on the beach, a walk in the woods, witness a fiery sunrise, or watching a magnificent sunset. For all of us, satisfying the soul is a way of finding inner peace, a calming sense of well-being that feels good deep, down into our being.

We seldom stop to realize that we *receive a great deal more than we give. By being grateful we satisfy the soul appreciate the richness of our lives. As we continue to nurture our inner being, we are able to openly express our feelings, give and receive love, keep an open mind, and see ourselves as we truly are. Gratitude unlocks and opens us to the fullness of life. Gratitude for the past brings peace today, and creates vision for tomorrow.*

Dozens of studies have demonstrated a link between spirituality and better health. Research has shown people with spiritual beliefs enjoy greater health and longevity. Spiritually active people have been shown to recover from illnesses more quickly and to cope better with stress. Prayer has been shown to bring forth a "relaxation response" that relieves stress and heightens the sense of well-being.

Multiple studies have documented the power of prayer. Everyday prayer can help us experience great spiritual heights when our hearts are touched by moments of exquisite beauty. These moments of grace may be rare of course, but they could capture our whole life and lift us from the mundane, giving us a fresh insight into all the lows in our life. People who make everyday prayer a habit had a heightened sense of well-being.

Satisfying your soul means doing what makes you feel happy, calm, and complete. It means living an authentic life and not playing a role. It means finding your life and living it.

There is so much to see, to learn, to give, to do in life as a way of satisfying the soul. Where should you start? It really doesn't matter, as long as you begin. Do something that you have always wanted to do, no matter what anybody else thinks or says. Take up piano, learn a foreign language, write, paint; the possibilities are endless. Skinny-dip. Spend a day at a nursing home. Make your own bread. Laugh out loud. Sing Karaoke. Dance the jig. Learn to sew. Be a mentor. Send someone a "thinking of you" card .Have your palm or tarot cards read. Rearrange all the furniture in your living room. Vote. Inspire someone. Get remarried. Be frivolous. Be a star. Plant a vegetable garden, and then eat what you grow. Change jobs. Give up being perfect. Change your mind. Let the phone ring. Write your memoirs. Make angels in the snow. Tell your children all about your life. Sit

in an empty church. Allow yourself to be

awestruck.   Break a tradition.   Trust yourself.   Make out like a

bandit. Give to the less fortunate.   Play with puppies. Sleep on satin sheets. Research a subject

you've always wanted to know about. Collect seashells. Start a conversation with a stranger. Get a

tattoo. Burn bridges to the troublesome parts and people of your life. Inhale. Beat the odds. See a

rodeo. Comfort the afflicted. Buy someone a present for no reason at all. Soak in a hot tub. Write

thank-you notes when it isn't necessary. Show up. Slow up. Smell the flowers, the cooking, and the

rain. Bake brownies. Move. Keep a journal. Put 20 bucks in a slot machine. Buy a lottery ticket.

Share the wealth. Tell the truth, especially when it's hard. Expect nothing.   Stand the test of time.

Love more than once.   Make a wish upon a star. Witness a miracle. Enjoy the moment without

expecting it to last.   Take part in heaven on earth.   Accept mortality, but live forever. Fall asleep

counting your blessings. Celebrate your life every day for no reason, and for every reason.   Explore

your own potential and your own life's possibilities. Sometimes it is good and invigorating to try

something different or new. It's easy for all of us to go on as we always have because it requires no

effort. But once you stop trying to make an effort, you start looking and acting old. How long has it

been since you took yourself off, on your own, to somewhere you've never been before- to

somewhere totally new even for an hour? It is a mini-adventure and a wonderful chance to keep your

mind and eyes open. People look but often don't see. Notice the architecture on the road you drive

every day. When you go strolling through the garden section of your favorite store, stop to pay close

attention to the seasonal flowers and foliage.   Go to a different mall or park and just sit and observe.

Find a café and spend some leisure time watching people. Go to a different neighborhood or part of

the city and absorb the different atmosphere. You never need to be bored when there are other

people around. Being an explorer in your own life doesn't have to cost you a penny. You can explore without going too far from home and discover a world you have really seen.

Another powerful way of nurturing the soul and deepening our spirit is to adopt an attitude of gratitude. Inspirational and motivational experts encourage us to incorporate a gratitude and appreciation practice into our lives. This helps bring us into a very positive state of awareness and receiving. The words "please and thank you," were taught to us as children. We teach our children the tradition and it will continue to be taught throughout generations.

The words "thank you" are important; but why? A quote from Melodie Beatte, freelance author and journalist states: "gratitude unlocks the fullness of life. It turns what we have into enough and more. It turns denial into acceptance, chaos into order, and confusion into clarity. It turns problems into gifts, failures to success, the unexpected to perfect timing and mistakes into important events. Gratitude makes sense of our past, brings peace for today and creates a vision for tomorrow."

The simple phrase "thank you," the gestures or even the thoughts you think in giving appreciation, showing gratitude, are powerful and magnetic ways of attracting, manifesting and receiving abundance and happiness into your life. Imagine giving a friend wonderful gifts but that friend never say thank you, never shows gratitude or send a card of appreciation. It would not be a surprise if you suddenly stopped giving your friend gifts. And so it is with the universe as you give thanks for your health, family, your job, your talents, life events, joys and opportunities in your life, you attract positive vibrations that create and bring more abundance, harmony and balance to you.

Read, think about and practice the following quotes and see how they will affect your life.

Anthony Robbins states, "when you are grateful fear disappears and abundance appears."

Brian Tracy says, "develop an attitude of gratitude and give thanks for anything that happens to you, knowing that every step forward is a step toward achieving something bigger and better than your current situation."

"The deepest craving of human nature is the need to be appreciated."

William James.

The following reports from research studies emphasize the powerful effects of gratitude.

According to Rind, B., and Borda, P. 1995. Effect of Servers "Thank You"

and Personalization on Restaurant Tipping. Journal of Applied Social Psychology.

They found that restaurant patrons gave bigger tips when their servers wrote "Thank You" on their checks.

According to Kashdan, T. B., Uswatte, G., Julian, T. 2006, Gratitude and Hedonic and Eudaimonic Well-Being in Vietnam War Veteran s Behavior Research and Therapy.

"Although gratitude is something that everyone can experience, some people seem to feel grateful more often than others. People who tend to experience gratitude more frequently than do others, also tend to be happier, more helpful, giving and less depressed than their

less grateful counterparts."

So, what can you do to express more gratitude and attract more harmony, peace, love and abundance into your life?

Simple Ways to Express Gratitude :

Make a list of the things you are thankful for in the physical, spiritual, emotional, financial, social and educational aspects of your life.

As you go through this list you will amaze yourself of the increase in positive energy and gratefulness that you will feel.

The best things in life are free- sunrise and sunsets, a beautiful moonlit night, the sky, the rain, a magnificent mountain range- stop, look, listen and feel the wonders of Mother Nature and express your gratitude.

Write a thank you note to a friend or family member expressing your gratitude and appreciation for having them in your life. This will create a higher level of positive energy in your relationship.

A phone call to a friend expressing appreciation or encouragement can make a difference in their day and in your own.

Show encouragement and appreciation to the people you interact with on a daily basis. A co-worker, the banker, the clerk at checkout counter or your neighbor.

Share your abundance with others. This is a way of telling the universe thank you and uplifting the life of others.

Feelings of gratitude comes from the heart, as you open your heart and express gratitude more positive energy, love and peace will come into your life. As we appreciate the good in our lives and focus on it, the exhilarating positive vibrations that we give off serve to draw more of the same to us. Understanding and using this concept can greatly enhance our life by supercharging our sense of accomplishment and self-worth

One of the most powerful ways to focus on appreciation is at night, at the end of our day. When we are winding down from all the activity of the day and our mind starts to quiet, then we can effectively tune in to our inner thoughts and body rhythms. We can then clearly reflect on what we are grateful for from that particular day.

Here are a few suggestions:

1) Affirmations - Write a few positive gratitude statements about those events and people that inspired you that particular day. These can be very specific or they can be general. You can focus in on people or events, or just pick up on the uplifting emotions of the day. You can even repeat these affirmations in the morning as a continuation of the good-feeling state of mind from the previous night.

2) Journaling – Take a few minutes to write an entry in a journal or notebook. Or just write a "gratitude note." You don't need to write an entire volume — just a few clear sentences about those especially fulfilling moments in your day that caught the gratitude feeling in your heart!

3) Gratitude in the Mirror – In his book "The Success Principles" Jack Canfield suggests a uniquely empowering gratitude practice which is done with mirror work. Look at yourself in the mirror and have an upbeat conversation with yourself. Appreciate yourself with a series of statements reflecting on your day and your accomplishments, both small and large.

I try to do this right before bed, so it helps get my subconscious mind into a positive and serene place. For example, I might say "Sheryl, I appreciate all you have done today. You wrote two articles today. You posted to your blog. You worked on building your Reiki practice. You set three new goals. You had that extremely healthy salad for lunch. Even though you really didn't feel like it, you went to work out at the gym and you felt great afterward. You cooked your husband's favorite meal." Then — and this is essential — express love for yourself! This may feel and seem odd at first, but if you can get into this, it is a very effective self-empowerment tool.

4) Gratitude Focus at Bedtime – If mirror work does not quite resonate with you, then try a few gratitude moments right before bed, or even in bed, before you drift off to sleep. Take this time to reflect on your day. Choose activities and accomplishments that were meaningful to you.

Appreciate the goodness of your day. Even if you feel it was not the easiest of days, FIND those bright spots and center in on those. Even if you had a demanding day on the job, but you finished a project, or moved along on one, or helped someone else solve a problem or accomplish something, celebrate that. Congratulate yourself on any goals you attained. Replay any special family or friend moments that bring a smile to your heart. As with the Gratitude in the Mirror suggestion, make sure to appreciate yourself too. Thank yourself for just being you and for doing the best that you can with the knowledge and life understanding that you have. Then, let yourself be lulled to sleep in this positive state of mind.

Affirmation, Attitude, Action ; to help bring in the daily appreciation:

- *Today was filled with inspiring people, joyful experiences and heartwarming memories.*

- *It is easy for me to recall all the beautiful aspects of my day — and I am gratefu*

- *In this place of appreciation, I look forward to tomorrow and welcome joyful experiences into*

my life.

Martin Seligman, a researcher and teacher at the University of Pennsylvania, is considered the father of positive psychology. He developed an inventory, the VIA (which stands for Values In

Action) Survey of Character Strengths, which allows individuals to explore character traits and rate their personal strengths and aspects of happiness. He noticed that when an individual had an insufficient appreciation of good events, and an overemphasis of bad or unfortunate experiences, it greatly undermined their serenity, contentment and satisfaction with life.

Seligman conducted research with his students, using one of the exercises that Emmons and McCullough developed in their experimental investigations, namely, counting your blessings. When asked to write down five things for which they felt grateful for, once a week, for 10 weeks in a row, exciting results emerged. Students reported feeling less stressed, more content, optimistic and satisfied with their life. These were similar to findings of other researchers, which showed that participants who counted their blessings on a regular basis became happier as a result.

Even more interesting, when Dr. Seligman than asked his student to write gratitude letters to significant individuals in their lives, and conduct gratitude visits where they read those letters out loud to the recipients, it fostered not only increased feelings of joy, but also a closer meaning and pleasure derived from the relationship.

It would appear that counting our blessings on a regular basis can improve our moods and overall level of happiness and health, but expressing that appreciation to others will do so even more. And the good news is that noticing, appreciating and expressing our feelings for life's *little* blessings can produce just as much benefit as noticing the monumental moments.

So it certainly seems that developing a higher level of gratitude is emotionally, physically and mentally rewarding. **But, how do you increase your feelings of gratitude when nothing seems to be going right, or life presents great challenges and adversity?** Is it really possible to express gratitude when you are not feeling you have anything to be grateful for?

Although we may acknowledge gratitude's benefits, it can still feel difficult to feel grateful when we are going through a difficult time. That's why it makes so much sense to *practice* gratitude, in good times and bad. It may be human nat

And the most difficult way to strengthen our souls and our spirits is the practice of "letting go" and allowing what will be to be. Another way to phrase the same idea is "walking by faith and not by sight."

It is a very difficult idea to follow, but the freedom that comes with it is a gift to the soul.

Allowing can be either the most difficult thing to do, or the most freeing. For those of us who have control issues (*raising hand*) letting go and allowing the universe to work on our behalf is terrifying. W e've developed a belief that if we want something done right we have to do it ourselves. Leaving it to anyone else means it will probably be done poorly or not at all. Of course, such a belief only sets us up to receive exactly that outcome.

But not allowing goes even deeper than control issues. At its core, a resistance to allowing also reveals a bigger blockage: Lack of trust in the order of things.

In order to really allow, we need to be willing to trust that the universe knows what we want and can find the best possible way to bring it to us. We need to trust that it will all unfold with perfect timing.

We need to trust our own power as deliberate creators of our life paths. We need to trust that our intuition is strong enough to recognize when we're being led in a specific direction – and that we'll know which actions to take when the time is right.

All of this can be scary, really scary. In order to fully let go, we need to get comfortable with the idea of free-falling. Trusting our faith is like free-falling without a parachute. Free-falling without a parachute even though it appears we're heading straight for some jagged rocks. In that moment our firs t impulse might be to panic and do "something" to control the outcome.

But something amazing happens when we can muster the courage to let go, trust, and hold to the inner vision of what we want. A strong wind gusts up from underneath us and guides us to exactly where we want to be. Sometimes it guides us to something even better than what we thought we wanted. And we look back and laugh at how silly our fear and doubt seem when viewed through the clarity of hindsight.

Allowing, trusting, letting go is a gift and an opportunity. Letting go and allowing is an opportunity to refine our focus and tone our faith muscles. Every time we make a conscious decision to let go and allow, it becomes easier to do. We grow in confidence – both in ourselves and in the universe as a loving, supportive force.

It seems to be part of human nature to notice all that is wrong in our lives or that we lack, but if we give ourselves the chance on a regular basis to notice all of lives gifts and blessings, we can increase our sense of well-being, and create hope and optimism for the future—no matter what is going on.

Martin Seligman, a researcher and teacher at the University of Pennsylvania, is considered the father of positive psychology. He developed an inventory, the VIA (which stands for Values In Action) Survey of Character Strengths, which allows individuals to explore character traits and rate their personal strengths and aspects of happiness. He noticed that when an individual had an insufficient appreciation of good events, and an overemphasis of bad or unfortunate experiences, it greatly undermined their serenity, contentment and satisfaction with life.

Seligman conducted research with his students, using one of the exercises that Emmons and McCullough developed in their experimental investigations, namely, counting your blessings. When asked to write down five things for which they felt grateful for, once a week, for 10 weeks in a row, exciting results emerged. Students reported feeling less stressed, more content, optimistic and satisfied with their life. These were similar to findings of other researchers, which showed that participants who counted their blessings on a regular basis became happier as a result.

Even more interesting, when Dr. Seligman than asked his student to write gratitude letters to significant individuals in their lives, and conduct gratitude visits where they read those letters out loud to the recipients, it fostered not only increased feelings of joy, but also a closer meaning and pleasure derived from the relationship. Martin Seligman, a researcher and teacher at the University of Pennsylvania, is considered the father of positive psychology. He developed an inventory, the VIA (which stands for Values In Action) Survey of Character Strengths, which allows individuals to explore character traits and rate their personal strengths and aspects of happiness. He noticed that when an individual had an insufficient appreciation of good events, and an overemphasis of bad or unfortunate experiences, it greatly undermined their serenity, contentment and satisfaction with life.

It would appear that counting our blessings on a regular basis can improve our moods and overall level of happiness and health, but expressing that appreciation to others will do so even more. And the good news is that noticing, appreciating and expressing our feelings for life's *little* blessings can produce just as much benefit as noticing the monumental moments.

So it seems that developing a higher level of gratitude is emotionally, physically and mentally rewarding. **But, how do you increase your feelings of gratitude when nothing seems to be going right, or life presents great challenges and adversity?** Is it really possible to express gratitude when you are not feeling you have anything to be grateful for?

Although we may acknowledge gratitude's benefits, it can still feel difficult to feel grateful when we are going through a difficult time. That's why it makes so much sense to *practice* gratitude, in good times and bad. It may be human nature to notice all that is wrong or that we lack, but if we give ourselves the chance on a regular basis to notice all of lives gifts and blessings, we can increase our sense of well-being, and create hope and optimism for the future—no matter what is going on.

• We all know how short and transitory our life is: I don't mean what the statistical tables say about just how long we live, but how short it all is when we are alive, celebrating life together with those we love. We give a part of ourselves when we share, and each of us has something to share that no one else does. Savoring every minute of life creates moments where living becomes our soul's satisfaction.

• Poets, writers, and musicians aspire to heightened moments of awareness; times they feel they have something unique and inspiring to give to the world. Most creative people do what they do because there is something burning inside of them; creating is a way of life for them that satisfies their souls.

• We want to *feel the purpose of our lives. We want to know the reason that we are here. As Samuel Johnson so eloquently put it, "To improve the golden moment of* opportunity and catch the good that is within our reach is the *great art of life". And each of those moments feed the depths of our soul and deepen our appreciation for our lives.*

- Think about it. Look around and give thanks for all the blessings you have received. Do something spiritual, wonderful, crazy, or inspirational and satisfy the deepest needs of your soul.

Keep It Moving

Bibliography

1. Doress-Worters, Paula B.and Diana Laskin Siegal, *Ourselves, growing Older, Touchstone(* New York, New York 1987,1994)

2. Cohen, Gene D., *The Mature Mind: the positive power of the aging brain ;(Basic Books, ,* 2005)

3. Erwin, Kathie T., *Foundations of gerontology ;(P.A. Hutchison Publishing Company, 2006)*

4. , Chris and Henry S. Lodge M.D., *Younger next year; (Workman Publishing, New York*

2004)

    5. Croker, Richard, *The Boomer Century 1946-2046 ;(Springboard Press, , 2007),*

    6. Cooke-Kearney, Ann, *Change Your Mind, Change Your Body: Feeling good about yourself after 40; (Atria Books, , 2004),*

    7. Crandall, Susan, *Thinking about Tomorrow: reinventing yourself at Midlife ;(Warner Wellness,),*

    8. Levine, Robert M.D., *Aging with Attitude; Growing Older with dignity and Vitality,(Praeger Publishers, 2004),*

    9. Pilzer, Paul Zane, *The Wellness Revolution; How to Make a fortune in the Next Trillion dollar Industry, (John Riley&Sons, Inc., , 2002)*

    10. Null, , *Power Aging; The revolutionary program to control the Symptoms of aging Naturally,(New American Library, , 2003)Gary*

    11. Smith, Hyrum W., *The 10 Natural Laws of Successful Time and Life Management, (Warner Books, Inc., New York, 1994)*

    12. Gerzon, Mark, *Listening to Midlife, (Shambhala Publications, Boston Massachusetts, 1992*

    13. Hollis, James PhD., *Finding Meaning in the Second Half of Life, (Gotham Books, , 2005),*

    14. Davidson, Sara, *LEAP!, (Random House, , 2007)*

    15. Progrebin, Letty Cottin, *Getting Over Getting Older, (Little, Brown & Company, New York, 1996)*

    16. Dychtwald, Ken, Ph.D., *Age Power, (Penguin Putnam Inc., New York,1999)*

    17. Novelli, Bill, *50+, (St. Martin's Press, , 2006)*

    18. Haas, Robert, M.S., Eat to Win for Permanent Fat Loss, (Harmony Books, ,2000)

    19. Gaesser, Dr. Glenn A., *The Spark; A Revolutionary New Plan to get Fit and lose Weight, (Rodale Inc. ,,2001)*

    20. Schwalbe, Robert, PhD , *Sixty, Sexy, and Successful; A Guide for Aging Male Baby Boomers, (Praeger Publishers, , 2008) ,*

21. Cruise, Jorge, *8 Minutes in the Morning; Extra Easy Weight Loss*, (HarperCollins Publishers Inc., , 2004)

22. Lydon, M.D.,Christine, *Ten Years Thinner,*(Da Capo Press, , 2008),

23. Roulac, Ann Nichols, *Power, Passion & Purpose; 7 steps to Energizing Your Life*, (Green Island Publishing, Larkspur, , 2006)

24. , Robert J., PhD., *The Healthy Skeptic*, (of Press, , 2008)DavisUniversityCalifornia

25. Sansone, Leslie, *Walk Away the Pounds*, (Time Warner Book Group, , 2005)

26. Smith, Kathy, *Lift Weights to Lose weight*, (Warner Books, Inc., ,2001)

27. Stoddard, Alexandra, *Living a Beautiful Life*, (Random House, New York,1986)

28. Collin, Joan, *The art of Living Well; Looking good and Feeling Great*, (Sourcebooks Inc., , 2007),

29. Winter, Paul A., Book Editor, *The Civil Rights Movement*, (Greenhaven Press, Inc., , 2000),

30. Weil, Andrew, M.D., *8 Weeks to Optimal Health*, (Ballantine Publishing Group, New York, 1997)

31. Chopra, Deepak, M.D., *Ageless Body, Timeless Mind*, (Harmony Books, New York, 1993)

32. Gullo, Stephen P.,PH.D., *Thin Tastes Better*, (Carol Southern Books, ,

1995)

33. Balch, Phyllis, A., CNC, *Prescription for Dietary Wellness*, (Penguin Books, , 2003)

1. Torkos,Sherry and Wassef, Farid, *Breaking the Age Barrier,*(Penguin Books, , 2003),

2. Dyer, Wayne W., *Real Magic*, (HarperCollins Books, New York, 1989)

3. Wilson, Douglas, *Doug's rooms* ,(Clarkson/Potter Publishers, , 2004)

4. Fifield, Katherine, *Instant Style*, (In Style Books, , 2006)

5. Simontacchi, Carol, *Crazy Makers; How the Food Industry is destroying our brains and

Harming our children,(Penguin Putnam Inc., , 2000)

6. Stoddard, Alexandra, *Open Your Eyes, (HarperCollins, New York, 1998)*

7. Fuller, Kristi M., R.D. Editor, *Eating For Life, (Meredith Books, , 2001),*

8. Haas, Robert, M.S., *Eat to Win for Permanent Fat loss, (Random House Inc., , 2000)*

9. Breus, Michael, Ph.D., *Good Night; The sleep doctor's 4-week program to better sleep and better Health, (Penguin Group, New York, 2006)*

10. , James B., *Sleep Power,(Villard Books, New York, 1998)Maas*

11. Zhigang Sha, Dr., *Soul Wisdom ı (Heaven's Library Publication Corp., , 2007)*

12. Bazilian, Wendy, „ RD., *The Super Foods Rx Dieı, (Rodale, Inc., , 2008)DrPHMA*

13. Somers, Suzanne, *Slim & Sexy forever, The Hormone Solution for permaneni weight loss and Optimal Living, (Crown Publishers, , 2005)*

14. Brody, Jane, *Jane Brody' s Nutrition Book; guide to good eating for better Health and Weight Controı,(W.W. Norton & Company Inc. , 1981)*

15. Lipper, Jodi and Vincent, Cerina, *How to Eat Like a Hot Chick*, (, 2008),

16. Krupp, Charla, *How Not to Look Old*, (Springboard Press, , 2008)

17. Robinson, Chris, *The Core Connection*, (Simon Spotlight Entertainment, , 2009)

18. Westerterp, K.R., *"Diet Induced Thermogenesis"*, *"Nutrition& Metabolism (2004) 1:5*

19. Pratt, Steven, " *Super Health"*, (Penguin Group Inc., 2009)

20. Pratt, Steven and Meadows, Kathy, *"Super Foods"*, HarperCollins Publishers, 2005)